Prasanta Kumar Biswal
Prafulla Kumar Sahu

# ATORVASTATIN SELF-EMULSIFIED TABLETS FORMULATION AND EVALUATION

Prasanta Kumar Biswal
Prafulla Kumar Sahu

# ATORVASTATIN SELF-EMULSIFIED TABLETS FORMULATION AND EVALUATION

## SELF-EMULSIFIED DRUG DELIVERY SYSTEM

LAP LAMBERT Academic Publishing

**Imprint**
Any brand names and product names mentioned in this book are subject to trademark, brand or patent protection and are trademarks or registered trademarks of their respective holders. The use of brand names, product names, common names, trade names, product descriptions etc. even without a particular marking in this work is in no way to be construed to mean that such names may be regarded as unrestricted in respect of trademark and brand protection legislation and could thus be used by anyone.

Cover image: www.ingimage.com

Publisher:
LAP LAMBERT Academic Publishing
is a trademark of
Dodo Books Indian Ocean Ltd. and OmniScriptum S.R.L publishing group

120 High Road, East Finchley, London, N2 9ED, United Kingdom
Str. Armeneasca 28/1, office 1, Chisinau MD-2012, Republic of Moldova, Europe

ISBN: 978-620-5-52808-2

# ATORVASTATIN SELF-EMULSIFIED TABLETS FORMULATION AND EVALUATION


*Prasanta Kumar Biswal[1]*, Prafulla Kumar Sahu[2]*

[1]*Department of Pharmaceutics, Gayatri College of Pharmacy, Sambalpur, Odisha, India.*

[2]*Department of Pharmaceutical Analysis, School of Pharmacy, Centurion University of Technology and Management, Odisha, India.*

**<u>PREFACE</u>**

Due to a variety of factors, including poor drug solubility and absorption, many medication candidates fall short of their therapeutic effectiveness expectations. SEDDS, or self-emulsifying drug delivery systems, have received recognition for their capacity to improve the solubility and bioavailability of medicines that are not readily soluble. When SEDDS are placed into an aqueous phase while being gently stirred, they emulsify spontaneously to create fine oil in-water emulsions. SEDDS are available in soft or hard gelatin capsules for oral administration, and upon aqueous dilution, they produce fine, comparatively stable oil-in-water emulsions. SEDDS are typically prepared as liquid formulations, which have some drawbacks such as poor stability and portability, low drug loading, a limited number of dosage form options, irreversible drug/excipient precipitation, and the use of a large amount (30–60%) of surfactants that can irritate the gastrointestinal tract. To get around these drawbacks of liquid SEDDS, an alternate strategy called solid-SEDDS has been researched. One of the finest methods for obtaining free-flowing powders for compression into tablet dosage form, which might be referred to as self-micro-emulsified tablets is the adsorption of liquid self-micro-emulsified formulations on solid carriers (SMET).

Aiming to improve the stability and oral bioavailability of atorvastatin, present research intends to design and optimise the SMET formulation. The improved SMET will next be tested in rabbits for pharmacokinetic parameters as AUC, Cmax, Tmax, Vd, Ke, t1/2, and TCR. The study's objectives were met by the study's findings. By utilising the information already accessible on the study's subject, it can be said that the research's findings have added a new level of understanding to the fields of formulation creation and biopharmaceutical drug modification.

**ABBREVIATION**

| | | | | | |
|---|---|---|---|---|---|
| $(t_{1/2})_a$ | : | Absorption Half life | ICH | : | International Conference on Harmonization |
| $(t_{1/2})_e$ | : | Elimination Half life | IS | : | Internal Standard |
| ANOVA: | | Analysis Of Variance | IST | : | Isothermal stress testing |
| ATVN | : | Atorvastatin | $K_a$ | : | Absorption Rate Constant |
| $AUC_{0-\infty}$ | : | Area Under the Curve from Zero to Infinity | $K_e$ | : | Elimination Rate Constant |
| AUMC | : | Area Under the Momentum Curve | $K_{o/w}$ | : | Partition Coefficient |
| BCS | : | Biopharmaceutical Classification Systems | LC | : | liquid crystals |
| CCS | : | Cross Carmelose Sodium | MCC | : | Microcrystaline Cellulose |
| CI | : | Compressibility Index | MCT | : | Medium-chain triglyceride |
| $C_{max}$ | : | Maximum Plasma Drug Concentration | MRT | : | Mean Residence Time |
| CP | : | Cross Povidone | PEG | : | Polyethylene glycol |
| CPCSEA: | | Committee for Prevention, Control and Supervision of Experimental Animals | $pK_a$ | : | Dissociation Constant |
| CR | : | Controlled Release | PRESS | : | Predicted Residual Sum of Square |
| CV | : | Correlation of variance | PVP | : | Polyvinylpyrrolidone |
| $D_b$ | : | bulk density | RSD | : | Relative Standard Deviation |
| df | : | Degree of Freedom | RSM | : | Response Surface Methodology |
| $DR_{30}$ | : | % of drug release at 30 min | SEDDS | : | Self Emulsifying Drug Delivery Systems |

| DR$_5$ | : | % of drug release at 5 min | SELS | : | self-emulsified liquid system |
| DR$_{60}$ | : | % of drug release at 60 min | SMEDDS | : | Self-micro-emulsifying drug delivery systems |
| DSC | : | Differential Scanning Calorimeter | SS | : | Sum Square |
| D$_t$ | : | tapped density | S-SEDDS | : | Solid-SEDDS |
| DT | : | Disintegration Time | t$_{50}$ | | Times required for 50 % of drug release |
| F | : | Calculated Fischer's Ratio | t$_{80}$ | | Times required for 80 % of drug release |
| FDA | | US Food and Drug Administration | TCR | : | Total Clearance Rate |
| GIT | | Gastrointestinal tract | T$_{max}$ | : | Time to achieve maximum plasma drug concentration |
| HLB | | Hydrophilic lipophilic balance | V$_b$ | | bulk volume |
| HPMC | : | Hydroxy Propyl Methyl Cellulose | V$_d$ | : | Volume of Distribution |
| HR | | Hausner ratio | | | |

# CHAPTER 1

## INTRODUCTION

## Overview

About 60% of innovative drug candidates are poorly water soluble, causing low bioavailability, intra- and inter-subject variability, and dosage proportionality [1]. Surfactants, lipids, permeation enhancers, micronization, salt formation, cyclodextrins, nanoparticles, and solid dispersions are employed to address these challenges [1,2]. Recently, lipid-based formulations and self-emulsifying drug delivery systems (SEDDS) have received much attention to boost the oral bioavailability of lipophilic medications [3,4]. Self-emulsifying drug delivery systems increase the solubility and bioavailability of poorly soluble medications. SEDDS are isotropic mixtures of oils, surfactants, and co-solvents intended to improve the oral bioavailability of lipophilic drugs [5-9]. SEDDS emulsify spontaneously when added to an aqueous phase and gently stirred, resulting in fine oil-in-water emulsions. SEDDS come in soft or firm gelatin capsules that, when diluted in water, create fine, stable oil-in-water emulsions.

The stomach and intestines' GI motility agitates self-emulsifying formulations, allowing them to pass smoothly through the GIT. Small droplet size and disintegration give a large interfacial surface for effective medication absorption. SMEDDS form emulsions with droplet sizes less than 50 nm, while SEDDSs create emulsions between 100 and 300 nm [10,11]. SEDDSs are physically stable and easily made, unlike emulsions. These systems may boost the rate and extent of absorption for lipophilic medicinal compounds with dissolution rate-limited absorption [4]. LC and gel phases form during self-emulsification. Controlling the LC (liquid crystal) at the interface is critical for drug release from SEDDS.

## Solubility

Solubility is the greatest amount of a solute that may be dissolved at a particular temperature. Solubility is the ability of one substance to dissolve another. A solution has a solute and a solvent (the dissolved fluid). Solution is when a solute is totally dissolved in a liquid [12,13]. In solubilization, to dissolve a solute, the solvent must disrupt the solute's inter-ionic or intermolecular bonds. Solubility depends on particle size, temperature, pressure, solute and solvent type, molecular size, polarity, and polymorphs [14].

8

## Enhancing solubility

Dosage forms are evaluated based on their ability to transport active chemicals to the site of action in sufficient amounts to deliver the desired pharmacological response. Physiological availability, biologic availability, or bioavailability describe this dose form property. Bioavailability is the rate and degree of drug absorption into the systemic circulation. For convenience and stability, most drugs are manufactured into tablets or capsules [15-18]. Absorption of solid dosage forms involves tablet disintegration and release of solid drug particles, drug particle dissolution in aqueous gastrointestinal fluid, permeation of drug molecules from intestinal fluid through unstirred aqueous layer adjacent to mucosal surface, and drug permeation through mucosa and absorption.

Before being absorbed by the body, the active substance must be dissolved. Dissolution slows drug absorption from solid dose forms, especially if the drug is weakly soluble. Bioavailability and solubility determine pharmacological compounds' therapeutic efficacy. Solubility in the bloodstream is crucial to a drug's pharmacological effect. Nearly 40% of newly discovered chemical entities are weakly water-soluble medications, while only 8% have strong solubility and permeability.

## The Biopharmaceutics Classification System (BCS)

FDA created the Biopharmaceutics Classification System (BCS) to analyse oral medication products [20,21]. This method classifies medications into four classes based on biological membrane permeability and water solubility. A drug substance is deemed 'highly soluble' when the greatest dose strength is soluble in 250ml water or less over a pH range of 1 to 7.5, and 'highly permeable' when human absorption is 90% of an administered dose (in solution), based on mass balance or compared to an intravenous reference dose. 85% of a fast-dissolving tablet's medication must dissolve within 30 minutes. Most novel chemical entities are water-insoluble lipophilic compounds (Class II or IV). Developing medicinal medicines from such chemicals can be difficult.

**Class I** medicines are highly water-soluble, well-absorbed from the GI tract, and have favourable physicochemical qualities. Class I drugs are orally bioavailable.

**Class II** medicines are water-insoluble yet well-absorbed when dissolved. In vivo dissolving rate limits medication uptake. Due to formulation effects and in vivo factors, medicines in this family show varied absorption.

**Class III** medicines are water-soluble and don't easily pass bio membranes.

**Class IV** medications are water-insoluble and don't easily penetrate bio membranes.

**Solubility enhancement techniques:** The following section summarises strategies to improve medication solubility and absorption.

**Self-emulsified drug delivery system (SEDDS)**

**About self-emulsification**

Self-emulsification occurs when the entropy shift favouring dispersion is larger than the energy needed to enhance the dispersion's surface area [19]. The free energy of a typical emulsion creation is a function of the energy necessary to construct a new surface between the two phases (eq. 1).

$$\Delta G = \sum_i N_i \pi r_i^2 \sigma$$

Where, G is the free energy of the process (ignoring mixing), N is the radius of the droplets, and s is the interfacial energy. Over time, the emulsion's two phases will separate, reducing the interfacial area and free energy.

Conventional emulsifying agents generate a monolayer over emulsion droplets, reducing interfacial energy and preventing coalescence. Self-emulsifying systems require very little positive or negative free energy to generate an emulsion (then, the emulsification process occurs spontaneously). Emulsification with little energy input includes interfacial contraction. To emulsify, the interfacial structure must be shear-resistant. In prior work [22,23], it was postulated that emulsification ease could be related to how easily water penetrates LC or gel phases on droplet surfaces. According to Wakerly, adding a binary mixture (oil/nonionic surfactant) to water results in interface creation between the oil and aqueous-continuous phases, followed by solubilization of water inside the oil phase. This continues until the interface solubilization limit is reached. Aqueous penetration forms scattered LC phase. As water penetration continues, all material near the interface will be LC, the amount dependent on the binary mixture's surfactant concentration. Rapid water penetration into aqueous cores, helped by self-emulsification agitation, produces interface rupture and droplet production. Due to the LC interface around the oil droplets, these self-emulsified systems are resistant to coalescence [24]. Pouton et al. explored LC's role in emulsion formation. Craig et al. used particle size analysis and low frequency dielectric spectroscopy (LFDS) to evaluate the self-emulsifying properties of Imwitor 742/Tween 80 systems. Dielectric investigations showed a complex link between emulsion development and LC formation. The above technique noted that the medicine may modify emulsion properties by interacting with the LC phase. The link between spontaneous emulsification and LC formation isn't clear.

**Methodology**

Preliminary research are done to identify oil, a crucial ingredient in SEDDS. Oil, surfactant, and co-surfactant made up SEDDS. Different oils and surfactants determine medication solubility [25,26]. Prepare SEDDS with medication in oil and surfactant. The in vitro self-emulsification capabilities and droplet size analysis of these formulations are then examined. Pseudo-ternary phase diagram identifies self-emulsification zone. From these experiments, an improved formulation and its bioavailability are compared. The efficacy of oral absorption of the therapeutic ingredient from SEDDS depends on numerous formulation-related characteristics, such as surfactant concentration, oil/surfactant ratio, emulsion polarity, droplet size, and charge. Only very particular excipient combinations create self-emulsifying systems.

SMEDDS have smaller emulsion droplets, resulting in a clear or translucent solution. SMEDDS typically contain 40-60% w/w surfactant and hydrophilic co-solvents (e.g. propylene glycol, polyethylene glycols). They're called micro emulsion pre-concentrates since the micro-emulsion forms in water.

- The solubility of medication in the formulation as such and upon dispersion (for SEDDS),
- The rate of digestion (for formulations amenable to digestion), and perhaps
- The solubilization capability of the digested formulation.

**Oils**

Self-dispersing formulations use long- and medium-chain triglyceride (MCT) oils of varying saturation. Unmodified food oils are the most "natural" lipid carriers, but their inability to dissolve hydrophobic medicines and difficulties self-emulsifying reduces their usage in SEDDS [27]. Modified or hydrolyzed vegetable oils have helped these systems succeed. Formulate and physiological benefits. These excipients create good emulsification systems with non-ionic surfactants authorised for oral administration, although their breakdown products resemble intestinal digestion. Early self-emulsifying formulations preferred MCTs. They have improved fluidity, solubility, and self-emulsification, although they are less attractive than innovative semi-synthetic medium chain derivatives, which are amphiphilic compounds with surfactant characteristics. In such instances, lipophilic surfactant may replace hydrophilic oil [28]. Blending triglycerides with mono- and di-glycerides improves hydrophobic medication solubility.

**Surfactants [19-23]**

Non-ionic surfactants with a high hydrophilic lipophilic balance (HLB) were recommended for self-dispersing systems [19,20]. Ethoxylated polyglycolyzed glycerides and Tween80 are the most commonly utilised excipients. Natural emulsifiers are safer than synthetic ones and suggested for SDLF use, despite their low self-emulsifying potential. Non-ionic surfactants are less hazardous than ionic surface-active chemicals, however they can promote reversible intestinal wall permeability [23-29]. Amemiya et al. presented a fine emulsion with limited surfactant content (3 percent) to minimise toxicological issues associated with high surfactant concentration. Self-emulsifying formulations require 30 to 60% w/w surfactant to generate and maintain an emulsion in the GI tract. Surfactant can irritate the GI tract in excessive quantities. Each situation should examine the surfactant vehicle's safety. High HLB and hydrophilicity of surfactants are required for early generation of o/w droplets and/or rapid spreading of the formulation in aqueous environments, enabling strong dispersing/self emulsifying performance [30]. Amphiphilic surface active agents can dissolve and solubilize hydrophobic drugs. This is crucial for preventing precipitation in the GI lumen and keeping medication molecules soluble for efficient absorption. Higher surfactant and co-surfactant/oil ratios generate self-microemulsifying formulations (SMEDDS).

**Co-solvents**

Self-emulsifying systems require high surfactant concentrations (typically over 30% w/w) [22,31]. Organic solvents suited for oral administration (ethanol, PG, PEG, etc.) may aid dissolve hydrophilic surfactant or medication in lipid base. Such systems may demonstrate some advantages over earlier formulations when integrated in capsule dosage forms, since alcohol and other volatile co solvents in conventional self-emulsifying formulations migrate into soft gelatin, or hard, sealed gelatin capsules, precipitating the lipophilic drug [32]. Alcohol-free formulations may have limited lipophilic drug solubility. With more cosurfactant, drug release increased.

**Factor Affecting SEDDS**

a) Concentration of drug: High-dose drugs aren't ideal for SMEDDS unless they're very soluble in at least one component, particularly the lipophilic phase.

b) Solubility of drug in oily phase affects SMEDDS's ability to solubilize drugs. If surfactant and co-surfactant solubilize more, precipitation may occur.

c) Polarity of lipid phase affects medication release from microemulsion. HLB, chain length, fatty acid unsaturation, hydrophilic part molecular weight, and emulsifier concentration determine droplet polarity.

## Advantages of SEDDS

a) Oral bioavailability increases dosage reduction.

b) Timely medication absorption profiles.

c) Selective targeting of drug(s) towards specific absorption window in GIT.

d) Drug(s) protection from stomach acid.

e) Reduced variability considering food influences.

f) Drug protection.

g) Solid or liquid doses.

h) In SEDDS, the lipid matrix interacts with water to generate a fine o/w emulsion. The emulsion droplets transfer the dissolved medication to the gastrointestinal mucosa. Many medications presented in SEDDS improve bioavailability and C max.

i) Fine oil droplets empty quickly from the stomach and facilitate extensive medication dispersion throughout the digestive system, minimising discomfort.

j) SEDDS is easier to create and scale up than solid dispersion, liposomes, nanoparticles, etc.

k) SEDDS can provide peptides for GIT enzymatic hydrolysis.

l) Polymer in SEDDS prolongs drug release.

## SEDDS disadvantages

Lack of adequate in vitro models for assessing self-emulsified drug delivery systems (SEDDS) and other lipid-based formulations is a challenge [33,34]. Traditional dissolve procedures don't work because these formulations depend on digestion. In vitro models modelling duodenum digestion have been constructed. Before evaluating its strength, this in vitro model needs more work. Further research will be based on in-vitro in-vivo correlations, therefore prototype lipid-based formulations must be produced and tested in vivo.

## SEDDS Applications

1. **Solubility and bioavailability:** SEDDS increases the solubility of Class- drugs (low solubility/high permeability) by bypassing the dissolution process. Ketoprofen, a

moderately hydrophobic (log P 0.979) NSAID, has a high propensity for stomach irritation during longterm therapy. Due to its limited solubility, sustained-release ketoprofen releases incompletely. Vergote et al. (2001) observed full drug release from nano-crystalline ketoprofen sustained-release formulations. Preparing matrix pellets of nano-crystalline ketoprofen, sustained release ketoprofen microparticles and formulations, floating oral ketoprofen systems, and transdermal ketoprofen systems can provide sustained release, boost bioavailability, and decrease gastrointestinal irritation. Nano-crystalline or enhanced solubility pharmacological forms may face production, stability, and economic issues. SEDDS-formulated Ketoprofen solves this problem. This formulation increases medication solubility and reduces stomach discomfort. Gelling agent in SEDDS prolonged Ketoprofen release.

In SEDDS, the lipid matrix interacts with water to generate a fine o/w emulsion. The emulsion droplets transfer the dissolved medication to the gastrointestinal mucosa. Many medicines presented in SEDDS improve bioavailability and Cmax.

2. **Anti-biodegradation:** Self-emulsifying drug delivery systems can reduce degradation and enhance absorption for medicines with low solubility and GI tract degradation. Many medications are destroyed in the body via acidic stomach PH, enzymatic or hydrolytic breakdown, etc [35]. When pharmaceuticals are in SEDDS, the liquid crystalline phase may act as a barrier between the drug and the degrading environment. Acetylsalicylic acid (Log P = 1.2, Mw=180) declines in the GI tract because it hydrolyzes to salicylic acid in acidic conditions. When the medicine was formulated in a GalacticlesTM Oral Lipid Matrix System (SEDDS formulation), it had a better plasma profile than the reference formulation. . The GalacticlesTM Oral Lipid Matrix System formulation improves the oral bioavailability of undegraded acetylsalicylic acid by 73%. This shows SEDDS can protect medicines from GI breakdown.

3. **Biopharmaceutical:** Lipids or meals can increase the bioavailability of weakly water-soluble drugs [36-39]. Although incompletely understood, lipids may increase bioavailability via several putative pathways, including:

   a. **Gastric transit slows, increasing dissolution time:** The presence of lipids in the GI tract promotes the production of bile salts (BS) and endogenous biliary lipids including phospholipids (PL) and cholesterol (CH), resulting to the creation of BS/PL/CH intestinal mixed micelles and an increase in the GI tract's solubilization capacity. Intercalation of supplied (exogenous) lipids into these

BS structures directly (if sufficiently polar) or subsequent to digestion swells the micellar structures and increases solubilization capacity.

    **b. Stimulating intestinal lymphatic transport:** For lipophilic medicines, lipids may boost lymphatic transport and bioavailability directly or indirectly by reducing first-pass metabolism.

    **c.** Certain lipids and surfactants may attenuate intestinal efflux transporters, as demonstrated by the p glycoprotein efflux pump, and diminish enterocyte-based metabolism.

    **d.** Various combinations of lipids, lipid digestion products, and surfactants increase GI tract permeability. Passive intestinal permeability isn't a major barrier to the bioavailability of most poorly water-soluble and lipophilic medicines.

    **e.** Such compositions form a fine oil-in-water emulsion with gentle agitation from gastrointestinal motility. SES enhances plasma level–time profile repeatability. Physiological mechanisms have been proposed to explain the effect of oils on the absorption of water-insoluble compounds, including altered gastrointestinal motility, increased bile flow and drug solubilization, increased mucosal permeability, enhanced mesenteric lymph flow, and increased lymphatic absorption of water-insoluble drugs and bioavailability of hydrophobic compounds.

### *Solid self-emulsifying delivery system*

Solidification procedures: Capsule filling is the simplest and most frequent method for encapsulating liquid or semisolid oral SE formulations [40,41].

Semisolid compositions require four steps:

a) Heating semisolid excipient 20°C above melting point

b) Active ingredients (with stirring)

c) Melt capsules and

d) Room-temperature cooling.

Two-step method for liquid formulations:

a) Capsule-filling.

b) Banding or micro spray sealing capsule body and cap.

**Spray-drying**

This approach mixes lipids, surfactants, medication, and solid carriers before spray drying. Solubilized liquid is atomized into droplets. The droplets are put into a drying chamber, where the volatile phase (e.g., emulsion water) evaporates, forming dry particles. Tablets or capsules can be made from these particles [42]. The atomizer, temperature, airflow pattern, and drying chamber design depend on the product and powder.

**Solid-carrier adsorption**

Adsorption of liquid SE formulations to solid carriers produces free-flowing powders. Simple adsorption involves adding liquid formulation to carriers and blending. The powder can be immediately packed into capsules or combined with excipients before tableting. Adsorption improves content uniformity. Up to 70% (w/w) SEDDS can be adsorbed onto appropriate carriers. Solid carriers can be microporous inorganic substances, high-surface-area colloidal inorganic adsorbents, cross-linked polymers, or nanoparticle adsorbents, such as silica, silicates, magnesium trisilicate, magnesium hydroxide, talcum, crosspovidone, cross-linked sodium carboxymethyl cellulose, and cross-linked polymethyl methacrylate.

**Melt granulation**

Melt granulation combines powders by melting or softening a binder at low temperatures. Melt granulation is a 'one-step' operation, since liquid addition and drying are removed. It's also a solvent alternative. Impeller speed, mixing duration, binder particle size, and viscosity determine granulation. Melt granulation was utilised to adsorb SES (lipids, surfactants, medicines) onto solid neutral carriers (mainly silica and magnesium aluminometa silicate).

**Spheronization/melt extrusion**

Melt extrusion offers high drug loading (60%) and content consistency. Extrusion is the process of driving a raw material with plastic qualities through a die under controlled temperature, flow, and pressure. Extruder aperture size determines spheroid size. Pharmaceutical companies utilise extrusion–spheronization to generate uniform-sized spheroids (pellets). Extrusion–spheronization process steps:

a) Dry combining active components and excipients to make a powder; wet massing with binder

b) Spaghetti-like extrusion

c) Spheronization of the extrudate

d) Drying Sifting for size and coating (optional).

**S-SEDDS Dosage Form**

**Dry emulsion**: Dry emulsions are granules that self-emulsify in vivo or in water. Dry emulsions help make tablets and capsules. Dry emulsions are made by rotary evaporation, freeze-drying, or spray drying oil/water (O/W) emulsions containing a solid carrier (lactose, maltodextrin, etc.) in the aqueous phase. By rotational evaporation with heavy mineral oil and sucrose, Myers and Shively made solid state glass emulsions. Emulsifiable glasses don't need surfactant.

Slow cooling and amorphous cryoprotectants provide the highest stabilising effects in freeze-drying, but heat treatment before thawing lowers them. Spray drying is used to make dry emulsions. Spray-drying the O/W emulsion removed the aqueous phase. Newly discovered enteric-coated dry emulsion formulation could be used for oral delivery of peptide and protein medicines. This lyophilized formulation included a surfactant, vegetable oil, and pH-responsive polymer. Cui et al. made dry O/W emulsions by spreading liquid emulsions over a flat glass, then drying and powdering them.

**Self-emulsifying capsules:** After taking capsules containing liquid SE, micro emulsion droplets form and distribute in the GI tract to absorption sites. If the micro emulsion irreversibly separates, drug absorption won't improve. For this, sodium dodecyl sulphate was added to SE. Super saturable SEDDS was meant to prevent drug precipitation by producing and maintaining a supersaturated condition in-vivo. This system's lower surfactant reduces GI side effects. In addition to liquid filling, solid or semisolid liquid SE components can be added to capsules (adsorbents, polymers, and so on). Solid PEG matrix is one example. Solid PEG did not affect the drug's solubility or self-microemulsification in water.

Self-emulsified capsules improve patient compliance compared to parenteral administration. LMWH, used to treat venous thromboembolism, was only accessible parenterally. So, rigid capsules were made for oral LMWH therapy. LMWH was distributed in SMEDDS, and the mixture was solidified using three adsorbents: micro porous calcium silicate (FloriteTM RE), magnesium aluminium silicate (NeusilinTM US2), and silicon dioxide (SylysiaTM 320) [19,43]. These solids were encapsulated. In another work, these adsorbents were used to make SE tablets of gentamycin, which was only available in injectable or topical formulations.

**Sustained-release self-emulsifying tablets:** Combinations of lipids and surfactants show promise for creating SE tablets. Nazzal and Khan studied the effect of processing parameters (colloidal silicates—X1, magnesium stearate mixing time—X2, and compression force—X3) on tablet hardness and CoQ10 dissolution. Face-centered cubic design optimised (X1 = 1.06 percent, X2 = 2 min, X3 = 1670 kg). Patil et al. created a gelled SEDDS to reduce the amount of solidifying excipients needed for solid dosage forms. In their investigation, colloidal silicon dioxide (Aerosil 200) was used as a gelling agent for oil-based systems, lowering the amount of hardening excipients and slowing medication release. Schwarz's patent reveals that SE pills prevent unwanted effects. Incorporating indomethacin (or another hydrophobic NSAID) into SE pills may boost its GI mucosal membrane penetration, lowering GI haemorrhage. In these experiments, SES contained glycerol monolaurate and Tyloxapol™ (a copolymer of alkyl phenol and formaldehyde).

**Self-emulsifying SR pellets:** Pellets, a multiple unit dose form, have numerous advantages over conventional solid dosage forms, such as manufacturing flexibility, reducing intra- and inter-subject plasma profile variability, and limiting GI irritation without lowering drug absorption.

Combining pellets and SEDDS by SE pellets is intriguing. Serratoni et al. [45,46] produced SE controlled release pellets by integrating pharmaceuticals into SES that boosted their release rate and then covering pellets with a water-insoluble polymer that decreased drug release. Extruded/spheronized pellets contained water-insoluble model pharmaceuticals (methyl and propyl parabens); SES contained mono diglycerides and Polysorbate 80. According to another publication, SE sustained release matrix pellets can be made using glyceryl palmitostearate and glyceryl behenate.

**Solid dispersions:** Solid dispersions could boost the dissolution rate and bioavailability of weakly water-soluble medicines, however manufacturing and stability issues occurred. Serajuddin said SE excipients [47] potentially solve these problems. These excipients may enhance the absorption of weakly water-soluble medicines compared to PEG solid dispersions and may be placed directly into hard gelatin capsules in the molten state, eliminating the need for milling and blending before filling. Gelucire144/14, Gelucire1 50/02, Labrasol1, Transcutol, and TPGS (tocopheryl polyethylene glycol 1000 succinate) are common SE excipients.

**SEL beads:** Patiland Paradkar examined loading SES into micro channels of porous polystyrene beads (PPB) via solvent evaporation. Copolymerizing styrene and divinyl benzene creates PPB with internal void structures. They're inert, pH- and temperature-stable, and humidity-resistant. This research found that PPB might solidify SES at high SES-to-PPB ratios. Bead size and pore architecture of PPB control loading efficiency and in vitro drug release from SES-loaded PPB.

**Sustained-release self-emulsifying microspheres:** Zedoaryturmeric oil (ZTO), a traditional Chinese medication, has tumor-suppressing, antimicrobial, and antithrombotic properties. You et al. developed solid SE sustained-release microspheres utilising quasi emulsion–solvent diffusion. The ratio of hydroxyl propyl methylcellulose acetate succinate to Aerosil 200 controls ZTO release. Rabbits given these microspheres orally had a bioavailability of 135.6 percent compared to liquid SEDDS.

**Self-emulsifying nanoparticles:** SE nano particles are produced using nano particle methods. One is solvent injection. In this process, lipid, surfactant, and medicines are melted and dropped into a stirring solvent [47,48]. SE nano particles were filtered and dried. These nano particles (100 nm) have a 74% drug loading efficiency.

**Self-emulsifying suppositories:** Some researchers found that SEDDS increased GI and rectal/vaginal adsorption 60. Oral glycyrrhizin hardly achieves therapeutic plasma concentrations, but vaginal or rectal SE suppositories can [49]. Glycyrrhizin was combined with C6–C18 fatty acid glycerol ester and macrogol ester.

**Self-emulsifying implants:** SE implant research has improved SEDDS's utility and application. Carmustine (BCNU) is used to treat malignant brain tumors [50]. Short half-life limited its usefulness. Loomis created bioresorbable, hydrophilic, cross-linkable copolymers. These copolymers have SE without an emulsifier. These copolymers are good prosthesis sealants.

**Reference**

1. Kommuru TR, Gurley B, Khan MA, and Reddy IK, Self-emulsifying drug delivery systems (SEDDS) of coenzyme Q10: formulation development and bioavailability assessment, Int J  Pharm, 2001, 212, 233-46.

2. Aungst BJ, Novel formulation strategies for improving oral bioavailability of drugs with poor membrane permeation or presys- temic metabolism, J Pharm Sci, 1993, 82, 979-987.

3. Humberstone AJ and Charman WN, Lipid-based vehicles for the oral delivery of poorly water soluble drugs, Adv Drug Del Rev, 1997, 25, 103-128.

4. Pouton CW, Formulation of self-emulsifying drug delivery systems, Adv Drug Del Rev, 1997, 25, 47-58.

5. Gursoy RN and Benita S, Self-emulsifying drug delivery systems (SEDDS) for improved oral delivery of lipophilic drugs, Biomed Pharmacother, 2004, 58, 173-82.

6. Gershanik T and Benita S, Self-dispersing lipid formulations for improving oral absorption of lipophilic drugs, Eur J Pharm Biopharm, 2000, 50, 179-88.

7. Shah NH, Carvajal MT, Patel CI, Infeld MH and Malick AW, Self- emulsifying drug delivery systems (SEDDS) with polyglycolized glycerides for improving in vitro dissolution and oral absorption of lipophilic drugs, Int J Pharm,1994, 106, 15-23.

8. Craig DQM, Lievens HSR, Pitt KG and Storey DE, An investigation into physico-chemical properties of self-emulsifying systems using low frequency dielectric spectroscopy, surface tension measure- ments and particle size analysis, Int J Pharm, 1993, 96,147-55.

9. Charman SA, Charman WN, Rogge MC, Wilson TD, Dutko FJ and Pouton CW, Self-emulsifying drug delivery systems: formulation and biopharmaceutic evaluation of an investigational lipophilic compound, Pharm Res, 1992, 9, 87-93.

10. Handbook of Chemistry and Physics (27th ed.), Cleveland, Ohio: Chemical  Publishing Co, 1943.

11. Greenwood GW, The Solubility of lipophyllic. Journal of Material Science, 1969, 4, 320–322.

12. Varshney S K, Zhong XF and Eisenberg A, Macromolecules, 1993, 26, 701-706.

13. Yalkowsky, Samuel H, Handbook of Aqueous Solubility Data, 1st Edition. Florida: CRC Press, 2003.

14. Horvath AL and Getzen FW, Halogenated Benzenes, Toluenes and Phenols with Water, Pergamon Press, Oxford, UK, 1985, Volume 20.

15. Shaw DG, Hydrocarbons in Water and Seawater, Part I, Pergamon Press, Oxford, UK, 1989, Volume 37.

16. Rosen MJ, Surfactants and Interfacial Phenomena (3rd ed.), Hoboken, New John Wiley and Sons, 2010.

17. Chen ML, Amidon GL, Benet LZ, Lennernas H and Yu LX, A theoretical basis for a biopharmaceutic drug classification: the correlation of in vitro drug product dissolution and in vivo bioavailability, Pharm Res, 2011.

18. Aungst BJ, Novel formulation strategies for improving oral bioavailability of drugs with poor membrane permeation or pre systemic metabolism, J Pharm Sc, 1993, 82, 979-986.

19. Wakerly MG, Pouton CW, Meakin BJ and Morton FS, Emulsification of vegetable oil-non-ionic surfactant mixtures, ACS Symp, Ser, 1986, 311, 242-255.

20. Becher P, Emulsions: Theory and Practice, Reprint, Krieger Pub, 1977.

21. Charman SA, Charman WN, Rogge MC, Wilson TD, Dutko FJ and Pouton CW. Self emulsifying drug delivery systems: formulation and biopharmaceutical evaluation of an investigational lipophilic compound, Pharm Res, 1992, 9, 87-93.

22. Acree Jr WE, Polycyclic Aromatic Hydrocarbons: Binary Non-aqueous Systems, Part I Solutes A-E, Oxford University Press, Oxford, UK, 1995, Volume4.

23. Hauss DJ, Fogal SE, Ficorilli JV, Price CA, Roy T, Jayaraj AA, Keirns JJ, Lipid-based delivery systems for improving the bioavailability and lymphatic transport of a poorly water-soluble LTB4 inhibitor, J. Pharm. Sci,1998, 87, 164–169.

24. Caliph SM, Charman WN, Porter CI, Effect of short-, medium- and long-chain fatty acid-based vehicles on the absolute oral bioavailability and intestinal lymphatic transport of halofantrine and assessment of mass balance in lymph-cannulated and non-cannulated rats, J. Pharm. Sci,2000, 89, 1073–1084

25. Jannin V, Musakhanian J, Marchaud D, Approaches for the development of solid and semi-solid lipid-based formulations, Adv Drug Deliv Rev, 2008, 60,(6),734–746.

26. Dong L, Shafi K, Wan J, Wong, In; Proceeding of the international symposium on controlled release of bioactive material, paris, 2003.

27. Keraliya RA, Patel C, Patel P, Keraliya V, Soni TG,. Patel RC and Patel MM, A new osmotic delivery system for controlled release of liquid formulation, Proceedings of the

International Symposiumon Controlled Release of Bioactive Materials, San Diego, (6) ,2001.

28. Cole ET, Challenges and opportunities in the encapsulation of liquid and semi-solid formulations into capsules for oral administration, Adv. Drug. Deliv. Rev, 2008, 60, 747–756.

29. Ito Y, Kusawake T, Ishida M and Tawa R, Oral solid gentamicin preparation using emulsifier and adsorbent, J control release, 2005,105, 23–31

30. Fabio C and Elisabetta C, Pharmaceutical composition comprising a water/oil/water double micro emulsion incorporated in a solid support.

31. Boltri L, Coceani N, DeCurto D, Dobetti L and Esposito P, Enhanced and modification of etoposide release from crospovidone particles loaded with oil-surfactant blends, Pharm Dev Technol, 1997, 2,373–381.

32. Venkatesan N, Yoshimitsu J, Ito Y, Shibata N, and Takada K, Liquid filled nanoparticles as a drug delivery tool for protein therapeutics, Biomaterials, 2005, 26, 7154–7163.

33. Seo A, Holm P, Kristensen HG, and Schæfer T, The preparation of agglomerates containing solid dispersions of diazepam by melt agglomeration in a high shear mixer, Int. J. Pharm,2003, 259, 161–171.

34. Gupta MK, Goldman D, Bogner RH, Tseng YC, Enhance drug dissolution and bulk properties of solid dispersions granulated with a surface adsorbent, Pharm. Dev. Technol,2001, 6, 563–572.

35. Seo A, Holm P, Kristensen HG, and Schæfer T, The preparation of agglomerates containing solid dispersions of diazepam by melt agglomeration in a high shear mixer, Int J Pharm, 2003, 259, 161–171

36. Gupta MK, Hydrogen bonding with adsorbent during storage governs drug dissolution from solid-dispersion granules, Pharm Res, 2002, 19, 1663–1672.

37. Verreck G, and Brewster ME, Melt extrusion-based dosage forms: excipients and processing conditions for pharmaceutical formulations, Bull Tech Gattefosse, 2004, 97, 85–95

38. Newton M, Petersson J, Podczeck F, Clarke A, and Booth S, The influence of formulation variables on the properties of pellets containing a self-emulsifying mixture, J Pharm Sci, 2001, 90, 987–995.

39. Booth SW, Clarke AP, Newton JM, and Godinho A, Formulation variables on pellets containing self-emulsifying systems, Pharm Tech Eur, 2005, 17, 29–33.

40. Newton JM, Bazzigialuppi M, Podczeck F, Booth S and Clarke A, The rheological properties of self-emulsifying systems, water and microcrystalline cellulose, Eur J Pharm Sci, 2005, 26, 176–183.

41. Tuleu C, Newton M, Rose J, Euler D, Saklatvala R, Clarke A, and Booth S, Comparative bioavailability study in dogs of a self-emulsifying-formulation of progesterone presented in a pellet and liquid form compared with an aqueous suspension of progesterone, J Pharm Sci, 2004, 93, 1495–1502.

42. Iosio T, Voinovich D, Grassi M, Pinto JF, Perissutti B, Zacchigna M, Quintavalle U and Serdoz F., Bi-layered self-emulsifying pellets prepared by co-extrusion and spheronization: influence of formulation variables and preliminary study on the in vivo absorption, Eur J Pharm Biopharm , 2008, 69,(2), 686-697.

43. Myers SL and Shively ML, Preparation and characterization of emulsifiable glasses: oil-in-water and water-in-oil-in-water emulsion, J Colloid Interface Sci, 1992, 149, 271–278

44. Bamba J, Cavé G, Bensouda Y, Tchoreloff P, Puisieux F and Couarraze G, Cryoprotection of emulsions in freeze-drying: freezing process analysis, Drug. Dev Ind Pharm, 1995, 21, 1749–1760.

45. Christensen KL, Pedersen GP and Kristensen HG, Technical optimization of redispersible dry emulsions, Int J Pharm, 2001, 212, 195–202.

46. Hansen T, Holm Per and Schultz Kirsten, Process characteristics and compaction of spray-dried emulsions containing a drug dissolved in lipid, Int J Pharm, 2004, 287, 55–66.

47. J. Bamba, G. Cavé, Y. Bensouda, P. Tchoreloff, F. Puisieux, and G. Couarraze, Cryoprotection of emulsions in freeze-drying: freezing process analysis, Drug Dev Ind Pharm, 1995, 21, 1749–1760.

48. Jang DJ, Jeong EJ, Lee HM, Kim BC, Lim SJ and Kim CK, Improvement of bioavailability and photo stability of amlodipine using redispersible dry emulsion, Eur J Pharm Sci, 2006, 28, 405–411

49. Toorisaka E, Hashida M, Kamiya N, Ono H, Kokazu Y, and Goto M, An enteric-coated dry emulsion formulation for oral insulin delivery, J Control Releas, 2005, 107, 91–96.

50. Cui FD, Hashida M, Kamiya N, Ono H, Kokazu Y, and Goto M, Preparation of redispersible dry emulsion using Eudragit E100 as both solid carrier and unique emulsifier, Colloid. Surf A: Physicochem. Eng. Asp, 2007, 07, 137–141.

# CHAPTER-2

## PROFILE OF DRUG AND EXCIPIENTS USED

### Atorvastatin for formulation of SEDDS

Hydrophobic drug i.e. Atorvastatin is a model drug for self-emulsifying solid drug delivery. It is an anti-hyperlipidaemic, statin group of lower the blood cholesterol level. Atorvastatin works by inhibiting HMG-CoA reductase, an enzyme found in liver tissue that plays a key role in production of cholesterol in the body [1-2].

### Regulatory Status

Bruce Roth at Parke-Davis Warner-Lambert initially synthesized atorvastatin in 1985. (now Pfizer). Pfizer and Ranbaxy agreed to delay the generic launch until November 2011. Pfizer called it Lipitor [3,4].

### Drug profile

### Structure

**Chemical structure of atorvastatin**

**IUPAC Name:** 3-phenyl-4-(phenylcarbamoyl)-5-(propan-2-yl)-1*H*-pyrrol-1-yl]-3, 5-dihydroxyheptanoic acid.

**Chemical Formula:** $C_{33}H_{35}FN_2O_5$

**Molecular Mass:** 558.64

**Physicochemical Properties** [3,4].

Melting point: 159.2-160.7 $^0C$

Solubility:  Atorvastatin calcium is very slightly soluble in distilled water, pH 7.4 phosphate buffer, and acetonitrile, slightly soluble in ethanol and freely soluble in methanol.

LogP: 5.7

PKa: 4.46

**Mechanism of Action**

Atorvastatin blocks HMG-CoA reductase. It's synthetic, unlike most others. HMG-CoA reductase catalyses the rate-limiting step in hepatic cholesterol production. Inhibiting the enzyme reduces de novo cholesterol production and increases LDL receptors on hepatocytes. This promotes hepatocyte LDL absorption, reducing blood LDL-cholesterol. Like other statins, atorvastatin decreases triglycerides and boosts HDL-cholesterol. In clinical studies, medications that restrict cholesterol uptake, such ezetimibe, complement those that block cholesterol production, like atorvastatin or simvastatin. [1,5-9]

**Pharmacokinetics** [10,11]

Atorvastatin has a Tmax of 1–2 hours after oral absorption. Absolute bioavailability is 14%; systemic availability for HMG-CoA reductase activity is 30%. High intestinal clearance and first-pass metabolism reduce atorvastatin's systemic availability. Food reduces Cmax (absorption rate) by 25% and AUC (absorption extent) by 9%, but it does not influence Atorvastatin's LDL-C-lowering efficacy. Evening doses diminish Cmax and AUC by 30%. atorvastatin's LDL-C lowering effectiveness is unaffected by administration timing. Atorvastatin is 98% protein-bound.

Activated ortho- and parahydroxylated metabolites, as well as beta-oxidation metabolites, are formed by cytochrome P450 3A4 hydroxylation. 70% of systemic HMG-CoA reductase activity comes from ortho- and parahydroxylated metabolites. Ortho-hydroxy metabolite glucuronidates. As a CYP3A4 substrate, inhibitors and inducers can increase or decrease plasma concentrations. In vitro, erythromycin, a CYP3A4 isozyme inhibitor, raised atorvastatin plasma concentrations. Atorvastatin inhibits 3A4.

Less than 2% of atorvastatin is excreted in urine. Hepatic and/or extrahepatic metabolism eliminates bile. No entero-hepatic recirculation appears. Atorvastatin's half-life is 14 hours. Due to active metabolites, HMG-CoA reductase inhibitory action has a half-life of 20–30h. Atorvastatin is a substrate of the intestinal P-glycoprotein efflux transporter, which pumps the medication back into the intestinal lumen.

Hepatic insufficiency affects plasma drug concentrations. Cmax and AUC quadruple in A-stage liver disease patients. Cmax and AUC rise 16-fold in B-stage liver disease patients. Geriatric patients' atorvastatin pharmacokinetics are 40% and 30% greater than in young adults. Healthy elderly patients have a better pharmacodynamic response to atorvastatin at any dose, therefore they may need lesser doses.

**Adverse Effects [12,13]**

Myopathy with elevated creatine kinase (CK) and rhabdomyolysis are rare (1%). Over 10% of patients get headaches. Weakness, insomnia, dizziness, chest pain, peripheral edoema, rash, abdominal discomfort, constipation, diarrhoea, dyspepsia, flatulence, nausea, urinary tract infection, arthralgia, myalgia, back pain, arthritis, sinusitis, pharyngitis, bronchitis, rhinitis, infection, flu-like syndrome, allergic response.

**Excipients used for the experiments**

***LINOLEIC ACID***

**Synonyms [14]:** Emersol 310; Emersol 315; leinoleic acid; 9-cis,12-cis-linoleic acid; 9,12-linoleic acid; linolic acid; cis,cis-9,12-octadecadienoic acid; Pamolyn; Polylin No. 515; telfairic acid.

**Chemical Name and CAS Registry Number**: (Z,Z)-9,12-Octadecadienoic acid [60-33-3]

**Empirical Formula and Molecular Weight:** $C_{18}H_{32}O_2$ , 280.45

**Structural Formula:**

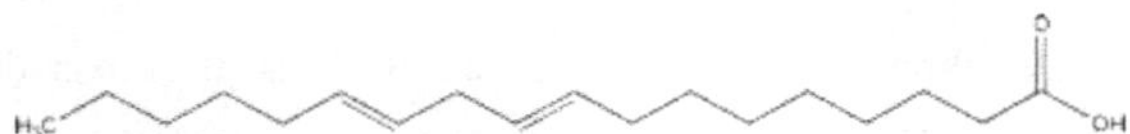

**Functional Category:** Dietary supplement; emulsifying agent; skin penetrant.

**Applications in Pharmaceutical Formulation or Technology**

Linoleic acid is utilised in topical transdermal, oral, cosmetic, and aqueous microemulsion formulations. It's employed in parenteral emulsions and oral food supplements.

**Description:** Linoleic acid occurs as a colorless to light-yellow-colored oil.

**Typical Properties:**

**Boiling point:** 230.8 C at 16 mmHg

**Density:** 0.9007 g/cm

**Iodine value:** 181.1

**Melting point**: 58C

**Refractive index** : 1.4699

**Solubility** Freely soluble in ether; soluble in ethanol (95%); miscible with dimethylformamide, fat solvents, and oils.

**Stability and Storage Conditions:** Linoleic acid is sensitive to air, light, moisture, and heat. It should be stored in a tightly sealed container under an inert atmosphere and refrigerated.

**Incompatibilities:** Linoleic acid is incompatible with bases, strong oxidizing agents, and reducing agents.

**Method of Manufacture:** Linoleic acid is obtained by extraction from various vegetable oils such as safflower oil

**Safety:** Linoleic acid is widely used in cosmetics and topical pharmaceutical formulations, and is generally regarded as a nontoxic material. On exposure to the eyes, skin, and mucous membranes, linoleic acid can cause mild irritation.

**Handling Precautions:** Observe normal precautions appropriate to the circumstances and quantity of material handled. Gloves and eye protection are recommended.

**Regulatory Status:** GRAS listed. Approved for use in foods in Europe and the USA.

### *CROSCARMELLOSE SODIUM*

**Nonproprietary Names: BP:** Croscarmellose Sodium; **JP:** Croscarmellose Sodium; **PhEur**: Croscarmellose Sodium; **USP-NF:** Croscarmellose Sodium

**Synonyms [14]:** Ac-Di-Sol; carmellosum natricum conexum; crosslinked carboxymethylcellulose sodium; Explocel; modified cellulose gum; Nymcel ZSX; Pharmacel XL; Primellose; Solutab; Vivasol.

**Chemical Name and CAS Registry Number:** Cellulose, carboxymethyl ether, sodium salt, crosslinked [74811- 65-7]

**Functional Category**: Tablet and capsule disintegrant.

**Applications in Pharmaceutical Formulation or Technology:** It is used in oral pharmaceutical formulations as a disintegrant for capsules tablets, and granules. Croscarmellose sodium should be added in both the wet and dry stages of the process (intra-

and extra granularly) so that the wicking and swelling ability of the disintegrant is best utilized. Croscarmellose sodium at concentrations up to 5% w/w may be used as a tablet disintegrant, although normally 2% w/w is used in tablets prepared by direct compression and 3% w/w in tablets prepared by a wet-granulation process.

**Description:** Croscarmellose sodium occurs as an odorless, white or grayish- white powder.

**Typical Properties:**

**Acidity/alkalinity** pH = 5.0–7.0 in aqueous dispersions.

**Bonding index** = 0.0456

**Density (bulk)** = 0.529 g/cm$^3$ for Ac-Di-Sol

**Density (tapped)** = 0.819 g/cm$^3$ for Ac-Di-Sol

**Density (true)** = 1.543 g/cm$^3$ for Ac-Di-Sol

**Stability and Storage Conditions**

Croscarmellose sodium is stable, but hygroscopic. A direct-compression tablet formulation using croscarmellose sodium as a disintegrant revealed no difference in medication dissolution after 14 months at 308 C. Croscarmellose sodium should be kept cool and dry. Disintegrants like croscarmellose sodium may be less effective in wet-granulated or direct-compressed tablets containing hygroscopic excipients like sorbitol. Strong acids, soluble iron salts, aluminium, mercury, and zinc are incompatible with croscarmellose sodium.

**Safety:** It's harmless and nonirritant. Large dosages of croscarmellose sodium may have a laxative effect, however solid dosage formulations are unlikely to cause difficulties.

**Handling Precautions:** Observe safeguards suitable to the material and situation. Eye protection is suggested for croscarmellose sodium.

*MALTOSE*

**Nonproprietary Names:** JP: Maltose Hydrate; USP-NF: Maltose

**Synonyms [14]:** Advantose 100; Finetose; Finetose F;4-O-aD-glucopyranosyl-b-D- glucose; 4-(aD-glucosido)-D-glucose; malt sugar; maltobiose; Maltodiose; Maltose HH; Maltose HHH; Sunmalt; Sunmalt S.

**Chemical Name and CAS Registry Number:** 4-O-a-D-Glucopyranosyl-b-D-glucopyranose anhydrous [69-79-4] 4-O-a-D-Glucopyranosyl-b-D-glucopyranose monohydrate and [636353-7]

**Empirical Formula and Molecular Weight:** $C_{12}H_{22}O_{11}$, 342.30 (anhydrous); $C_{12}H_{22}O_{11}.H_2O$, 360.31 (monohydrate)

**Structural Formula:**

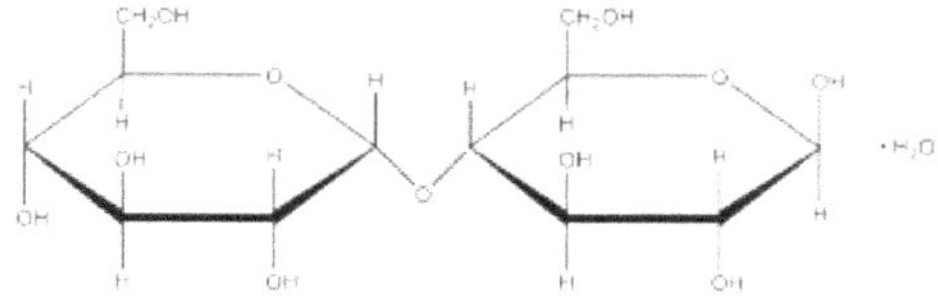

**Functional Category**: Sweetening agent; tablet diluents.

**Application:** Maltose is commonly used in food and pharmaceuticals. Maltose is a sugar used in parenteral medicines, especially for diabetes patients. Crystalline maltose is utilised in chewable and non-chewable direct-compression tablets.

**Description:** Maltose occurs as white crystals or as a crystalline powder. It odorless and has a sweet taste approximately 30% that of sucrose.

**Typical Properties**

*Acidity/alkalinity* pH = 4.5–6.5 for a 10% w/v aqueous solution.

*Angle of repose* = 37.18 for Advantose 100.

*Density (bulk)* = 0.67–0.72 g/cm³ for Advantose 100.

*Density (tapped)* = 0.73–0.81 g/cm³ for Advantose 100.

*Melting point* =120–1258C.

**Stability and Storage Conditions:** Maltose should be stored in a well-closed container in a cool, dry place.

**Incompatibilities:** Maltose may react with oxidizing agents. A Maillard-type reaction may occur between maltose and compounds with a primary amine group, e.g. glycine, to form brown-colored products.

**Method of Manufacture:** Maltose monohydrate is prepared by the enzymatic degradation of starch.

**Safety:** Maltose is used in oral and parenteral pharmaceutical formulations and is generally regarded as an essentially nontoxic and nonirritant material.

**Handling Precautions:** Observe normal precautions appropriate to the circumstances and quantity of material handled. Eye protection, rubber or plastic gloves, and a dust respirator are recommended. When heated to decomposition, maltose emits acrid smoke and irritating fumes.

## POLY VINYL PYRROLIDONE

**IUPAC Name :**Polyvinylpyrrolidone

**Other names [14]:** PVP, Povidone, Polyvidone Poly[1-(2-oxo-1-pyrrolidinyl)ethylen] 1-Ethenyl-2-pyrrolidon homopolymer 1-Vinyl-2-pyrrolidinon-Polymere Copovidone PNVP

**Identifiers**: CAS number          9003-39-8

**Properties:**

Molecular formula      : $(C_6H_9NO)_n$

Molar mass          : 2.500 - 2.5000.000 $g \cdot mol^{-1}$

Appearance          : white to light yellow, hygroscopic, amorphous powder

Density          : 1.2 g/cm³

Melting point          : 150 - 180 °C (glass temperature)

Properties          : PVP is soluble in water and other polar solvents. It absorbs up to 40% of its weight in atmospheric water when dry. It wets well and forms films easily in solution. It's a good coating or coating additive.

**Uses:** The monomer is extremely toxic to aquatic life.

**Medical:** The polymer PVP expanded trauma victims' blood plasma. PVP is a binder in many medicinal tablets; when combined with iodine, it forms the disinfectant povidone-iodine. It's utilised in solutions, ointments, pessaries, liquid soaps, and surgical washes. It's called Betadine. Pneumothorax (fusion of the pleura because of incessant pleural effusions).

**Safety:** This compound has various FDA-approved uses [13] and is typically harmless. PVP/povidone allergies have been reported.

## *TWEEN 80*

**Structural formula:**

**IUPAC name:** Polyoxyethylene (80) sorbitan monooleate

**Other names [14]:** Polyoxyethylene (80), sorbitan monooleate, (x)-sorbitan mono-9-octadecenoate poly(oxy-1,2-ethanediyl), Alkest TW 80, Tween 80, POE (80) sorbitan monooleate.

**Properties**

| | |
|---|---|
| *Molecular Formula* | : $C_{64}H_{124}O_{26}$ |
| *Molar mass* | : 1310 g/mol |
| *Appearance* | : Amber colored viscous liquid |
| *Density* | : 1.06-1.09 g/mL, oily liquid |
| *Boiling point* | : > 100°C |
| *Solubility in water* | : Very soluble |
| *Viscosity* | : 300-500 centistokes (@25°C) |
| *Main hazards* | : Irritant |

**Uses:** It is also used as an excipient in various European and Canadian influenza vaccinations. Some mycobacteria include a lipid-degrading enzyme. When added to Tween 80 and phenol red, they modify the colour of the solution, which is used to identify a strain's phenotypic.

## *POLYETHYLENE GLYCOL*

**Synonyms [14]:** Carbowax; Carbowax Sentry; Lipoxol; Lutrol E; PEG; Pluriol E; polyoxyethylene glycol.

**Empirical Formula:** $HOCH_2$ $(CH_2\ O\ CH_2)_m$ $CH_2\ OH$ (Where, m represents the average number of oxyethylene groups, n is a number m in the previous formula. Alternatively, the general formula $H\ (OCH_2\ CH_2)_n\ OH$ may be used to represent polyethylene glycol,

**Functional Category:** Ointment base; plasticizer; solvent; suppository base; tablet and capsule lubricant.

**Applications in Pharmaceutical Formulation:** Parenteral, topical, ophthalmic, oral, and rectal formulations. It's been employed in biodegradable controlled-release polymeric matrices. Polyethylene glycols can stabilise emulsions when combined with additional emulsifiers. Soft gelatin capsules use water-miscible polyethylene glycols. By absorbing gelatin moisture, they may harden the capsule shell.

**Solubility:** Polyethylene glycols dissolved in acetone, alcohols, benzene, glycerin, and glycols. Solid polyethylene glycols are soluble in acetone, dichloromethane, 95% ethanol, and methanol, but insoluble in fats, fixed oils, and mineral oil.

**Stability and Storage Conditions:** Chemically stable in air and solution, polyethylene glycols with a molecular weight below 2000 are hygroscopic. Polyethylene glycols don't support microbial development or get rancid. Polyethylene glycols should be kept in cool, dry containers. Liquids are stored in stainless steel, aluminium, glass, or lined steel.

**Incompatibilities:** All grades can exhibit some oxidizing activity owing to the presence of peroxide impurities and secondary products formed by autoxidation. Liquid and solid polyethylene glycol grades may be incompatible with some coloring agents. The preservative efficacy of the parabens may also be impaired owing to binding with polyethylene glycols. Plastics, such as polyethylene, phenolformaldehyde, polyvinyl chloride, and cellulose-ester membranes (in filters) may be softened or dissolved by polyethylene glycols. Migration of polyethylene glycol can occur from tablet film coatings, leading to interaction with core components.

**Safety:** Nontoxic and nonirritant. Low-molecular-weight glycols are toxic. Glycols are low-toxic. Topically applied polyethylene glycols may sting mucous membranes. Urticaria and delayed hypersensitivity reactions are reported. Patients with renal failure, extensive burns, or open wounds should use polyethylene glycol-containing topicals with caution.

## *MICROCRYSTALLINE CELLULOSE*

**Non-proprietary Names:** BP: Dispersible Cellulose; PhEur: Microcrystalline Cellulose; USP-NF: Microcrystalline Cellulose

**Synonyms [14]:** Avicel, cellulosum microcristallinum , carmellosum natricum; colloidal cellulose.

**Chemical Name:** Cellulose

**Functional Category:** Dispersing agent, stabilizing agent, suspending agent, thickening agent.

**Applications in Pharmaceutical Formulation or Technology:** Microcrystalline cellulose produces thixotropic gels for medicinal and cosmetic applications. Less than 1% solids create fluid dispersions, while 1.2+% solids create thixotropic gels. Used in nasal sprays, lotions, oral suspensions, emulsions, creams, and gels.

**Solubility:** Practically insoluble in dilute acids and organic solvents.

**Stability and Storage Conditions:** Moisture should not be exposed to hygroscopic microcrystalline cellulose. Stable at pH 3.5–11. Cool, dry storage recommended. Keep cool.

**Incompatibilities:** Microcrystalline cellulose is incompatible with strong oxidizing agents.

**Safety:** It is regarded as a non-toxic and non-irritant material.

**References**

1. Lennernas H, Clinical pharmacokinetics of atorvastatin, J Clin Pharmacokinet, 2003, 42, 1141–1160.

2. Kumar KM and Anil B, Biopharmaceutics drug disposition classification system, An extention of biopharmaceutics classification system, International Research Journal of Pharmacy, 2012, 3(3), 5 – 10.

3. The Merck Index, An encyclopedia of Chemicals, Drugs, and Biologicals, (14th ed.) Neil MJO, Editor Merck and Co. Inc, White house station, NJ, USA, 2006, 864 – 865.

4. Remington, The science and practice of pharmacy, (21th ed.) Lippincott Williams and Wilkins,2006, 1368-1369.

5. Malhotra HS and Goa KL, Atorvastatin; an updated review of its pharmacological properties and use in dyslipidaemia, J Drugs, 2001, 61, 1835–1881.

6. Srinivasa R, Prasad T, Mohanta GP and Manna PK, An overview of statins as hypolipidemic drugs, Int J Pharm Sci Drug Res, 2011, 3(3), 178-183.

7. Tamargo J, Caballero R, Gómez R, Núñez L, Vaquero M and Delpón E, Lipid-lowering therapy with statins, a new approach to antiarrhythmic therapy, Pharmacol Therap, 2007, 114, 107–126.

8. Zhang L, Zhang S, Jiang H, Sun A, Zou Y and Ge J, Effects of statin treatment on cardiac function in patients with chronic heart failure: A meta-analysis of randomized controlled trials, J Clin Cardiol, 2011, 34(2), 117–123.

9. Pichandi S, Pasupathi P, Raoc YY, Farook J, Ambika A and Ponnusha BS, The role of statin drugs in combating cardiovascular diseases. Int J Cur Sci Res, 2011, 1(2), 47 – 56.

10. Hamelin BA and Turgeon J, Relevance for the pharmacology and clinical effects of HMG-CoA reductase inhibitors, J Trends in Pharmacol Sci, 1998, 19, 26-37.

11. Lau YY, Okochi H, Huang Y and Benet LZ, Pharmacokinetics of atorvastatin and its hydroxy metabolites in rats and the effects of concomitant rifampicin single doses: Relevance of first – pass effect from hepatic uptake transporters, and intestinal and hepatic metabolism, Drug Met and Disp, 2006, 34(7),1175 – 1181.

12. Law MR, Wald NJ and Rudnicka AR, Quantifying effect of statins on low density lipoprotein cholesterol, ischaemic heart disease, and stroke: systematic review and meta-analysis, Br Med J, 2003, 326, 1423–1427.

13. Prueksaritanont T, Subramanian R, Fang X, Ma B, Qiu Y and Lin JH, et al, Glucuronidation of statins in animals and humans: a novel mechanism of statin lactonization, Drug Metabol Disp, 2002, 30, 505-512.

14. Hand Book of Excipient, (5th ed.) volume, 1998.

# CHAPTER-3

## PREFORMULATION

### Introduction

As a historical phenomenon, preformulation emerged in the early 1960s. Before this, many stability assays simply reported the amount of medicine that was initially put into the dosage form (such as those in official Pharmacopoeia). The introduction of stability-indicating assays into pharmaceutical operations, however, began in earnest in the early 1960s [1]. It soon became evident, however, that preparations needed to be made before formation could begin; this marked the birth of what is now known as "Preformulation" within the pharmaceutical sciences.

A medicine must generally go through preformulation before being nominated for commercial development. Characterizing substances' solid and solution physicochemical properties is called preformulation [2]. The nature of the drug substance can be defined with the help of data gleaned from preformulation experiments. This data is then utilised as a guide when formulating a dosage form of a medicine with other pharmaceutical substances [3]. According to Akers's [4] definition, preformulation is "the essential testing that comprises all research enacted on a new therapeutic molecule to yield meaningful information for later formulation of a stable and biopharmaceutically acceptable drug dosage form." To put it simply, preformulation is the study of determining the physicochemical properties of potential pharmaceuticals. Preformulation can also refer to investigations done to determine optimal conditions for formulating the candidate medicine.

Preformulation studies aim to determine the best drug delivery system by selecting the most appropriate drug substance form, evaluating the drug's physical qualities, and learning as much as possible about the drug's stability under various situations [5]. Preformulation studies typically focus on the drug's solubility, molecular formula and molecular weight, density, flow property and compressibility, particle size distribution, partition coefficient, ionisation constant, preferred polymorphic form, preferred dissolution method (medium), stability, and compatibility with other compounds (excipients). In addition to these variables, many others are determined on an as-needed basis. Different medication molecules and dosage forms necessitate distinct research approaches.

In order to create solid selfemulsified drug delivery systems, Atorvastatin (ATVN) was used for this work as model pharmaceuticals. Atorvastatin has been on the market for some time, and its physicochemical features have been documented in the previous chapter. ATVN is categorised as a BCS (biopharmaceutical categorization system) class-II medication (High permeability, low solubility) [6-8].

Understanding the many pharmacological and physiochemical properties of atorvastatin is the focus of this section. A standard calibration curve will be constructed using samples of the drug's solubility and dissolution in numerous physiological buffers, allowing for the estimation of the drug's concentration in those media. The compatibility of the drug with the excipients used in the formulation of solid self-emulsified drug delivery systems is an important consideration.

**Experimental**

**Materials**

Samples of atorvastatin were provided by Pfizer Company Ltd and Macleods Pharmaceuticals Ltd, both of Mumbai, India. Qualigens in Mumbai, India was the source for the Microcrystalline Cellulose (MCC) 101, Cross Povidone (CP), Maltodextrin (MD), Cross Carmelose Sodium (CCS), Maltose, and PVP K-30F. A variety of chemicals, including oleic acid, span 40, tween 80, lineloic acid, polyethylene glycol (PEG) 400, sodium hydroxide, methanol, ethanol, and potassium dihydrogen phosphate, were acquired from S.D Fine chemical Ltd in Mumbai, India. Every other compound was of analytical quality.

During the course of the study, the following instruments were employed: Fourier transform infrared spectrometer (8400S, Shimadzu, Japan); differential scanning calorimeter (JADE DSC, PerkinElmer, USA); ultraviolet-visible spectrophotometer (UV-1601, Shimadzu, Japan); digital weighing balance (Contech instruments Ltd., Mumbai); digital ultrasonicating cleaner (Loba Chemie., Mumbai); hot air oven (Universal).

**Standard calibration curve of atorvastatin in methanol**

Diluting the main stock solution of ATVN (100μg/ml) with methanol yielded standard solutions of ATVN with concentrations ranging from 3 to 30μg/ml. The maximum concentration of the medication (max) was determined by scanning a standard solution (15 μg/ml) using a UV-Visible spectrophotometer between 190 and 400nm. The standard calibration curve of ATVN in methanol was generated by plotting the absorbance of the standard solutions at $\lambda_{max}$ vs their concentrations.

**Standard calibration curve of atorvastatin in phosphate buffer, pH 6.8**

Standard solutions of ATVN (5, 10, 15, 20, 25, 30 and 35µg/ml) were generated by diluting the main stock solution (100µg/ml) with phosphate buffer, pH 6.8. The maximum absorbance of the medication was measured by scanning a standard solution (20 µg/ml) with a UV-Visible spectrophotometer between 190 and 400 nm. Standard calibration curve of ATVN in phosphate buffer, pH 6.8 was generated by plotting the absorbance of the standard solutions at $\lambda_{max}$ versus their concentrations.

**Moisture content of Atorvastatin**

Karl Fischer moisture determination device was used to calculate the drug's relative humidity using the following method. [11]

**Standardization of Karl Fischer reagent**

Sodium tartarate (100 mg) and dehydrated methanol (20 ml) were mixed for 1 minute before being titrated against the Karl Fischer reagent to an electrometric end point [11]. To determine the water equivalent factor in milligrammes of water per millilitre of reagent, we used the following formula:

$$F = (2 \times 18.02 \times w) / 230.08 \times v \tag{1}$$

Where, 'F' is the water equivalent factor, 'w', weight in mg of dehydrated sodium tartarate, 'v', volume of Karl Fischer reagent (ml). The molecular weight of sodium tartarate is 230.08, and the Karl Fischer constant is 18.02.

**Sample analysis**

In order to titrate against the Karl Fischer reagent, a sample of the medication (50 mg) was agitated for 1 minute in around 75 ml of dehydrated methanol. Sum of reagent volume used (S) to reach an electrometric plateau. A product of 'S' and a water equivalent factor (F), i.e., the water content, was obtained.

$$\text{Water content} = S \times F \tag{2}$$

**Flow properties of Atorvastatin powder**

With the use of the angle of repose, compressibility index, and hausner ratio, we were able to evaluate the powder's flow qualities. The following procedure was used to ascertain the flow characteristics of ATVN powder that had been sieved through No. 100 mesh.

**Angle of repose of the powder**

The angle of repose was calculated using the funnel technique. To get the tallest possible cone, the powder was poured into a funnel that was raised vertically on the flat surface. An angle of repose ($\theta$) was determined by measuring the radius of the pile (r).

$$\theta = \tan^{-1}(h/r) \tag{3}$$

**Bulk density of the powder**

Apparent bulk density ($D_b$) was determined by pouring the drug powder into a graduated cylinder. The bulk volume ($V_b$) and weight of the powder (M) was determined. The bulk density was calculated using the formula.

$$D_b = V_b/M \qquad\qquad (4)$$

**Tapped density of the powder**

The measuring cylinder containing a known mass of powder was tapped for 100 times. The minimum volume ($V_t$) occupied in the cylinder and the weight (M) of the blend was measured. The tapped density ($D_t$) was calculated using the following formula,

$$D_t = V_t/M \qquad\qquad (5)$$

**Compressibility Index of the powder**

Compressibility index (CI), the simplest method for measuring powder flowability, is computed as follows:

$$CI = [D_t-D_b/D_t] \times 100 \qquad\qquad (6)$$

The value below 15% indicates a powder with good flow characteristics, whereas above 25% indicate poor flowability.

**Hausner ratio of the powder**

The Hausner ratio [12] is a non-direct measurement of particle flowability. The formula for determining this is as follows:

$$\text{Hausner ratio} = D_t /D_b \qquad\qquad (7)$$

Where, $D_t$ is tapped density and $D_b$ is bulk density, Lower Hausner ratio (<1.25) indicates better flow properties and vice versa [13].

**Melting point determination of atorvastatin**

Melting point of ATVN was determined by using capillary tube method.

**FT-IR spectroscopic study of atorvastatin**

With an FT-IR spectrophotometer (JASCO 5300) and potassium bromide discs, we were able to record ATVN's IR spectrum between 400 and 500 cm$^1$.

**Differential scanning calorimetric study**

In order to conduct thermal analysis of the medication, a differential scanning calorimeter (JADE DSC, PerkinElmer, USA) was employed. Atorvastatin (after being strained through a 60-mesh filter) was weighed directly in the DSC aluminium pan and scanned between 50 and 3000 °C in an airless nitrogen chamber. The medication was heated at a rate of 200°C per minute, and the resulting thermograms were studied for identification purposes.

**Isothermal stress testing for Atorvastatin**

Drug and various excipients (Table 1) were weighed directly into 4 ml glass vials (n = 2) and combined on a vortex mixer for 2 minutes in IST experiments [14-15]. To each vial, water (10% v/w) was added, and a glass capillary was used to combine the medication excipients (both the ends of which were heat sealed). Capillary was shattered but left inside the vial to avoid waste. The teflon-lined screw caps were used to seal each vial, and the vials were then placed in a hot air oven set at 50 °C for storage. Every so often, we checked these samples to see if they had developed an odd hue. After keeping the samples in the conditions listed above for 3 weeks, a quantitative analysis was performed using a UV-Visible spectrophotometer. Controls consisted of drug-excipient mixtures kept in the fridge without water.

**Table 1: Interpretation of functional groups of Atorvastatin in the FTIR spectrum.**

| Sr.No | $\upsilon$ (cm$^{-1}$) | Functional group assignment |
|---|---|---|
| 1. | 3524.26 | N-H stretching. |
| 2. | 3030.44 | Aromatic –CH stretching. |
| 3. | 2943.64 | Ali C-H Stretching |
| 4. | 1689.80 | C=O stretching. |
| 5.. | 1605.8-1451.8 | Aromatic C=C stretching. |
| 6. | 1070-1030 | S=O Stretching |
| 7. | 1410 | Aliphatic C-N stretching |

The samples for drugs like ATVN were prepared by adding 2 ml of methanol and ethanol to each vial. After 3 minutes of whirling in a vortex, the fluid was poured into a 100 ml volumetric flask. There were two rounds of rinsing with methanol and ethanol in order to get the right volume for each vial. After centrifugation, the samples' supernatants were filtered using 0.45 μm nylon membrane filters. Samples were diluted as needed before being tested in a UV-Visible spectrophotometer at 245 nm and 253 nm wavelength against a blank, and the drug content was calculated using a calibration curve created within the predicted range.

**Stability study of Atorvastatin in dissolution medium**

Six volumetric flasks containing atorvastatin (3, 5, or 10 μg/ml) in USP-recommended dissolution medium (25 ml of phosphate buffer, pH 6.8) were prepared and stored at room temperature for 96 hours. We took a 24-hour, 48-hour, 72-hour, and 96-hour samples from each flask and filtered them at 0.45 μm. ATVN sample UV absorbance was measured at 245 nm against blank, and the amount of unchanged drug was computed using calibration curves of the drug produced in the aforementioned solvents. It was calculated as a percentage of the original concentration.

**Result and Discussion**

**Characterization of the drug**

**Melting point determination**

The melting point of ATVN was found to be 122 $^0$C, which comply the reported value of the drug.

**UV spectrum of the drug**

The UV spectrum of atorvastatin used in current work is shown in Figure 1. The resulted spectrums comply the reported spectrum of the drug.

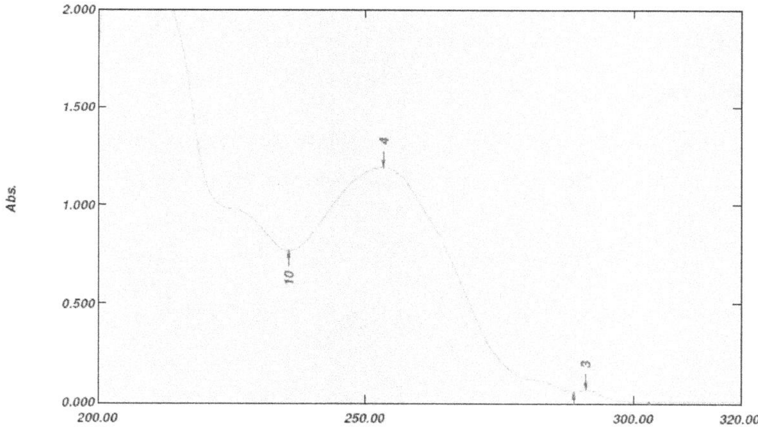


**Figure 1:`UV Spectrum of Atorvastatin**

**Differential Scanning Calorimetry**

The DSC thermogram of ATVN showed a sharp endothermic peak or peak of transition temperature ($T_{peak}$) at 121.63 $^0$C (Figure 2). The result again confirms the drug is ATVN.

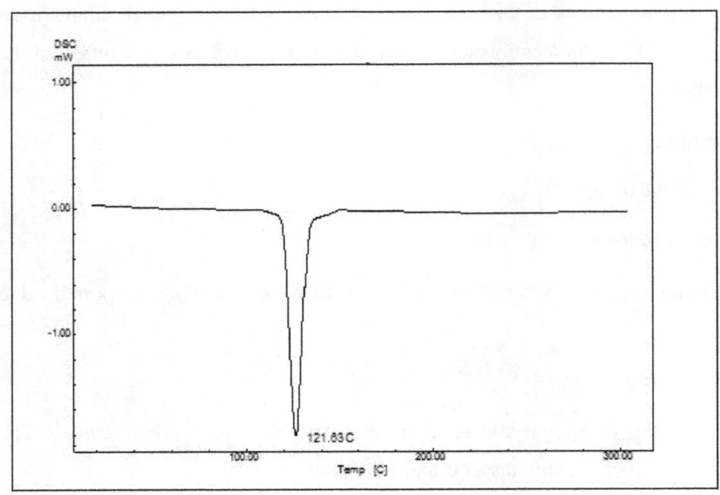

**Figure 2: DSC thermogram of Atorvastatin**

**FT-IR spectroscopic study**

The FT-IR spectrum of ATVN with its principal peak is shown in the Figure 3 and its interpretation is given in Table 1. This result complies with the structure of ATVN.

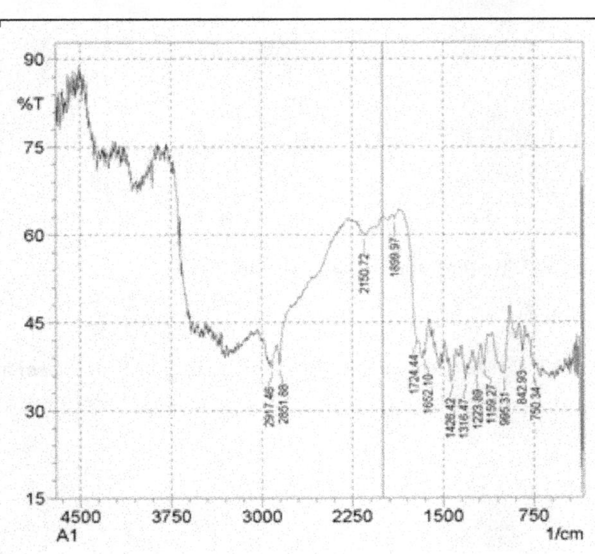

**Figure 3: FT-IR of Atorvastatin**

42

**Standard calibration curve**

Both medications' standard calibration curves were plotted in their appropriate organic solvents and dissolving media. Maximum absorption peak for ATVN in methanol was found to be at 245 nm, while for ATVN in phosphate buffer, pH 6.8, it was found to be at 259 nm, when scanned in the UV region. Beer-law Lambert's was shown to hold true for ATVN in methanol and phosphate buffer, pH 6.8 over concentration ranges of 0.3 to 30.0 µg/ml and 5.0 to 35.0 µg/ml. Figures 4 and 5 displayed the linear regression equation of concentration versus absorbance as well as the regression coefficient ($r^2$). The slope and intercept values of the linear calibration curve can be used to determine the concentration of the drug sample in different media, as shown by the $r^2$ values, which were all equal to 1.

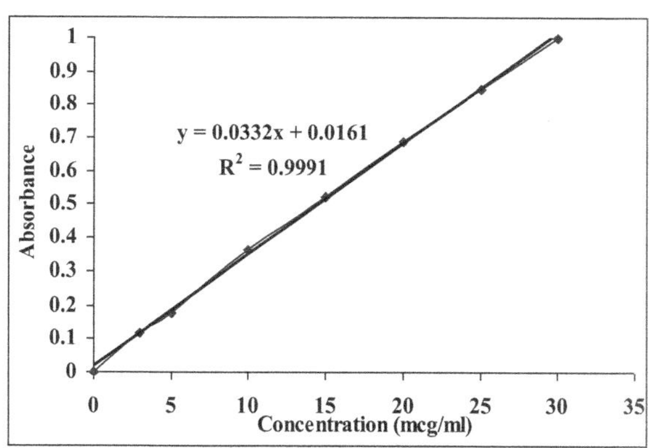


**Figure 4: Calibration curve of Atorvastatin in methanol** *(n=3)*

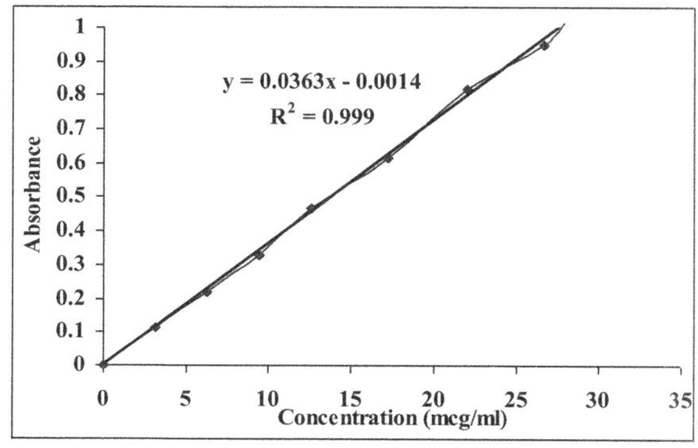


**Figure 5: Calibration curve of Atorvastatin in Phosphate buffer, pH 6.8** *(n=3)*

**Moisture content of Atorvastatin**

The determination of moisture present in the drug sample by Karl Fischer titration resulted a value of 0.6 %w/w and 0.3 %w/w respectively.

**Flow property of the drug**

The values for angle of repose, compressibility index and hausner ratio of Atorvastatin were found to be $49^0$, 36.48 % and 1.48 respectively.  The angle of repose $<30^0$ indicates free flowing material and $>40^0$ with poor flow properties. The compressibility index $<10\%$ indicates excellent flow properties and $>30$ with poor flow properties. Properties indicative of fluidity are those with a Hausner ratio between 1.00 and 1.11. The outcomes show that the medication has poor flow properties.

**Drug-excipient compatibility investigation using isothermal stress testing**

The quantitative findings of the IST tests performed on the excipients are shown in Table 2. The data demonstrates that some pharmaceutically active components are lost in drug-excipient mixtures while they are being stressed-stored. This means that the selected excipients can be added into atorvastatin self-emulsified tablet formulations.

**Table 2: Results of IST study of atorvastatin after 3 weeks of storage at stressed conditions**

| Samples | Ratios (drug-excipients) | % Drug remaining | |
|---|---|---|---|
| | | **Control samples** | **Stressed samples** |
| ATVN | — | 135± 0.48 | 116±0.84 |
| ATVN + Oleic acid | 1:1 | 134±0.51 | 122±0.62 |
| ATVN + Span40 | 1:1 | 122±0.43 | 111±1.78 |
| ATVN + Tween80 | 1:1 | 136±0.68 | 122±0.92 |
| ATVN + Cross povidone | 1:1 | 126±1.21 | 114±0.101 |
| ATVN + Maltodextrin | 1:1 | 109±1.28 | 99±1.98 |
| ATVN + Micro crystalline cellulose | 1:1 | 119±0.89 | 112±1.21 |

[a] Values expressed as average ± standard deviation.; [b] Drug excipient blends without added water and stored in refrigerator.

[c] Drug excipient blends with 10% (w/w) added water and stored at 50 $^0$C for 3 weeks.

**Stability study of atorvastatin in dissolution medium**

Dissolution media, such as phosphate buffer, pH 6.8, was used for the drug's stability testing. Table 3 shows the findings from the stability analysis. The results showed that after 96 hours of storage, there was no change in the initial concentration of the medication in the dissolving media. The medicine can be dissolved in the medium and appears to be stable there.

**Table 3: Stability study of atorvastatin in dissolution medium**

| Time interval (hr) | Concentration (µg/ml) | | |
|---|---|---|---|
| | Atorvastatin in Phosphate buffer, pH 6.8 | | |
| | Sample-1 | Sample-2 | Sample-3 |
| 0 | 30 | 20 | 10 |
| 24 | 29.64 ± 0.23 | 19.89 ± 1.04 | 9.96 ± 2.63 |
| 48 | 29.53 ± 1.28 | 19.84 ± 0.95 | 9.93 ± 1.94 |
| 72 | 29.26 ±1.11 | 19.79 ± 2.19 | 9.89 ± 1.82 |

**Conclusion**

As a result of this discovery, formulation development had to focus on enhancing the drug powder's poor flow characteristic. Atorvastatin's identity has been confirmed by its melting point, FTIR spectra, and DSC thermogram. According to the IST study, the proposed excipients selected for formulations are compatible with the medicine.

**References**

1. Carstensen JT, Introduction, In: Pharmaceutical Preformulation: Informa Health Care, New york, USA, 2006, 5-7.

2. Gerry S, Preformulation Predictions for Small Amount of Compound as an Aid to Candidate Drug Selection in: Mark G. (ed), Pharmaceutical Preformulation and Formulation: A Practical Guide from Candidate Drug Selection to Commercial Dosage Form: CRC Press Florida: USA, 2004, 21-22.

3. Loyd V and Allen JR, Dosage form design and development, Clinic Therapuet., 2008; 30: 2102-2111.

4. Akers MJ Preformulation testing of solid dosage forms. Methodology, management and evaluation, Can. J Pharm Sci, 1976, 1, 1-10.

5. Naazi SK The scope of preformulation studies In: Hand book of Preformulation: Chemical, Biological and Botanical drug: Informa Health Care, New york, USA, 2007, 57-58.

6. The Merck Index, An encyclopedia of Chemicals, Drugs, and Biologicals. 14th ed. Neil, M.J.O. Editor Merck & Co. Inc. White house station, NJ, USA (2006). P 864 – 865.

7. Remington. The science and practice of pharmacy. 21th ed. Lippincott Williams and Wilkins (2006). P 1368, 1369.

8. SRL inc, Biopharmaceutics Classification System (BCS), Therepeutic systeme research laboratory, available at http://www.tsrlinc.com/services/bcs/search.cfm, (Accessed 22/10/2012).

9. The Merck Index, An encyclopedia of Chemicals, Drugs, and Biologicals. 14th ed. Neil, M.J.O. Editor Merck & Co. Inc. White house station, NJ, USA (2006). P 924 – 825.

10. Remington. The science and practice of pharmacy. 21th ed. Lippincott Williams and Wilkins (2006). P 1373-1379.

11. Moisture content, Bulk density and Tapped density, In: United State Pharmacopoeia XXVII, NF-22, Asian edn, United State Pharmacopoeia Convention Inc, Rockville, USA, (2004) 2271-2272.

12. Lindberg N, Palsson M and Pihl A Flowability measurement of pharmaceutical powder mixtures with poor flow using five different techniques, Drug Dev Ind Pharm, 2004, 30: 785-791.

13. Levis SR and Deasy PB, Pharmaceutical application of size reduced grades of surfactant coprocessed microcrystalline cellulose, Int J Pharam, 2001, 230, 25-33.

14. Pani NR. and Nath LK, Development of controlled release tablet by optimizing HPMC: Consideration of theoretical release and RSM, Carbohydrate Polym, 2014, 104, 238-245.

15. Pani NR, Nath LK, Acharya S and Bhuniya B, Application of DSC, IST, and FTIR study in the compatibility testing of nateglinide with different pharmaceutical excipients, J Therm Anal Cal, 2012; 108: 219–226.

**CHAPTER 4**

**FORMULATING AND EVALUATING ATORVASTATIN SELF-EMULSIFIED TABLETS**

**Introduction**

Oral drug administration is convenient, however introducing poorly soluble medicines into systemic circulation is difficult [1]. Micronization, solid dispersion, and complexation are used to increase the oral bioavailability of poorly soluble medicines [2,3]. SEDDS, an isotropic mixture of oil, surfactant, co-surfactant, and drug (occasionally co-solvents), improves the solubility and bioavailability of poorly soluble medicines [4,5]. SEDDS emulsifies spontaneously in aqueous media to produce fine drug-in-oil emulsions with little agitation. SEDDS pills, tablets, and granules can be taken orally. When SEDDS are orally administered, the gastrointestinal tract's motility causes self-emulsification [6]. I dissolved drug; (ii) tiny droplet size gives a broad interfacial area for drug absorption. SEDDS are generally manufactured as liquids, which have low stability and mobility, low drug loading, few dosage form options, irreversible drugs/excipients precipitation, and high surfactant content (30–60%) that causes gastrointestinal irritation. Solid-SEDDS, an alternative to liquid SEDDS, has been investigated.

Solid-SEDDS are formed by solidifying liquid self-emulsifying components into powders/nanoparticles [7, 8]. Solid-SEDDS combine the benefits of SEDDS (i.e. solubility and bioavailability) with solid dose forms (e.g. low production cost, convenience of process control, high stability and reproducibility, better patient compliance.). Adsorption of liquid self-micro-emulsified formulations to solid carrier is one of the best ways to create free-flowing powders for tablet compression, called self-micro-emulsified macromolecules or self-micro-emulsified tablets (SMET). Physical and chemical attraction between liquid self-microemulsified formulation and adsorbing material affects microemulsion release rate from SMET. Using 23 factorial designs, the current study optimised the SMET adsorbent concentration. Response surface methodology is used to determine factor interactions for optimal SMET. Many pharmaceutical solid dose formulations use statistical optimization [9-12]. Using response surface approach, we designed, developed, optimised, and evaluated self-micro-emulsified atorvastatin tablets. During optimization, the primary, interaction, and

48

quadratic effects of formulation ingredients were studied. In-vivo rabbit pharmacokinetics determined SMET formulation bioavailability.

The eutectic interaction between a therapeutic entity and a eutectic agent could be used to develop improved lipid-based solid-state self-emulsified dosage forms to improve the stability and oral bioavailability of poorly soluble medicines. In this context, atorvastatin was chosen as a model pharmaceutical, and essential oils Oleic acid for atorvastatin was assessed as eutectic agent. Adsorption can be used to convert semisolid lipid-based self-emulsified medicinal dosage forms into solid tablets to increase formulation stability. Statistical optimization is utilised to improve tablet processing parameters to get desired results, and rabbits are used to determine in-vivo pharmacokinetic characteristics.

Current research aims to improve the stability and oral bioavailability of atorvastatin by developing SMET formulation. The atorvastatin SMET formulas were optimised using a 23-factorial design, with constituent concentrations as independent factors and tablet physiochemical properties as dependent variables. In rabbits, the improved SMET will be examined for pharmacokinetic characteristics (AUC, Cmax, Tmax, Vd, Ke, t1/2, TCR, etc.). As rabbit in-vivo pharmacokinetics data is similar to human studies, rabbits will be used in this study.

**Materials and Methods**

**Materials**

Gift samples of atorvastatin were generously provided by Pfizer Company Ltd, Mumbai, India. Products including Microcrystalline Cellulose 101, Cross povidone, Maltodextrin, and PVP K-30F were purchased from Qualigens in Mumbai, India. From S.D Fine chemistry Ltd in Mumbai, India, we ordered oleic acid, Span 40, Tween 80, sodium hydroxide, methanol, ethanol, and potassium dihydrogen phosphate. Other than what was needed for the experiment, all compounds employed were of a high enough purity for analytical usage.

**Drug-Excipient compatibility testing**

The drug-excipient compatibility testing was done with a differential scanning calorimeter and isothermal stress testing [11].

**Differential scanning calorimeter study**

Drug-excipient compatibility studies were performed with a differential scanning calorimeter on the excipients utilized in the formulation (JADE DSC, PerkinElmer, Waltham, MA, USA). The medicine and its excipients were sorted through an 80-mesh sieve before being weighed and scanned in a DSC aluminium pan between 50 and 300 degrees Celsius in a nitrogen environment at a heating rate of 20 degrees Celsius per minute.

**Isothermal stress testing study**

The research including isothermal stress testing was carried out in accordance with Pani et al [11] technique. As a quick recap, the medication and excipients were placed in glass vials and diluted with water at a concentration of 10% (w/w). The contents of each vial were secured with a Teflon-coated screw lid and kept at 50 degrees Celsius for up to 21 days. As a comparison, we used cold-stored, water-free drug-excipient mixes as the control. After 21 days, samples were taken from both the stressed and control groups and examined quantitatively with a UV-visible spectrophotometer.

**Preparation of Micro-emulsified Tablets**

**Self-emulsifying liquid preparation:** Weighing ATVN (23.1 percent w/w) and oleic acid (23.1 percent w/w) as oil basis at a ratio of 1:1into glass vial and mixing them at isothermal condition yielded the self-emulsified liquid system (SELS) of ATVN (370C). Two surfactants, Span 40 (2.69 percent w/w) and Tween 80 (2.69 percent w/w), were added to the oil mixture for a total of 30.04 percent w/w [13]. After that, a magnetic stirrer was used to blend the resulting emulsion into a clear solution. After that, the SELS sat out in the open air for 24 hours to cool down until they became a thick paste.

**Preparation of self-micro-emulsified tablets**

The adsorption-followed-by-compression phenomena was used to create the ATVN self-micro-emulsified tablets (SMET). In Table 2, we can see the SMET formulas. First, a semisolid waxy paste was made by grinding SELS paste with maltodextrin in a mortar and pestle. To obtain the dry emulsion-based granules, the mixture was ground with cross povidone for 1 minute. We then mixed the granules and MCC in a polybag for 5 minutes. Alcohol was pulverized with 12 mg of PVP and added to the adsorbed substance. Dried granules were obtained by placing wet granules through a 16 mesh sieve and drying them in a hot air oven at 450C. We mixed the dried granules with the leftover MCC and cross povidone. With an eight-station tablet compression machine (Lab press, Modle-1049, Ahmadabad, India) and an 8 mm die-punch set, the final blended mass was directly compressed.

**Characterization of self-emulsified granules**

Carr's approach (compressibility, angle of repose, and Hausner ratio) [10,14] was used to calculate the granular powder emulsion's flow characteristics.

**Characterization of self-micro-emulsified tablets**

Using the procedures outlined by Acharya et al., we analysed the physical properties of SMET, including its weight variation, drug content, thickness, hardness, friability, and disintegration tests. [11, 12]

**Measurements of Droplet Size and Turbidity**

To follow up on the tablet disintegration investigation, we measured the droplet size and turbidity of the emulsion we created using SMET. Centrifugation at 1000 rpm for 3 minutes separated the emulsion layer at supernatant from the adsorbed solid components present in the tablets from the medium containing the disintegrated tablets. The resulting emulsions were put through the following to determine droplet size and turbidity.

**Droplet size analysis**

To continue our research on tablet disintegration, we used SMET to make an emulsion and then measured its droplet size and turbidity. For 3 minutes at 1000 rpm, the solution containing the disintegrated tablets was centrifuged to separate the emulsion layer at supernatant from the adsorbed solid components present in the tablets. The following were applied to the generated emulsions to ascertain droplet size and turbidity:

**Turbidity measurement.**

Turbidity of the resultant emulsions given in nephlometric turbidity units (NTU) was measured using Digital Nephelo-Turbidity (Model 132, Systronics, Ahmedabad) with accuracy of ± 0.01 NTU with stray light less than or equal to 0.01 NTU. Turbidity measurement was carried out in 30 ml of emulsion.

**Dissolution study**

In order to continue our research on tablet disintegration, we used SMET to make an emulsion and then measured its droplet size and turbidity. The disintegrating tablets were centrifuged at 1000 rpm for 3 minutes, at which point the adsorbate layer and the emulsion layer were separated from the medium. The generated emulsions were placed through the following tests to quantify droplet size and turbidity.

**Design, statistics and optimization**

Using a $2^3$ factorial design with eight experimental trials, the optimal values for independent variables such as crosspovidone concentration (A; 50 and 70 percent), maltodextrin concentration (B; 100 and 120 percent), and microcrystalline cellulose concentration in tablets (C; 30 and 50 percent) were determined [9, 11, 12]. We chose as dependent responses the disintegration time (DT), the time needed for 50% drug release (t50), and the time needed for 80% drug release (t80). By analysing the outcomes of SMET formulations, research designs and response surface plots were generated in Design Expert software (Table 4). For the purpose of selecting the best fitting polynomial model, we computed statistical parameters including coefficient of variation (CV), regression coefficient ($R^2$), adjusted regression coefficient (adjusted $R^2$), F test, and P values. To determine which factors had statistically significant influences on which outcomes, an analysis of variance (ANOVA) was used. Measured answers from a $2^3$-factorial design were plugged into a mathematical equation that revealed the effects of each independent variable on the dependent variables.

$$Y = b_0 + b_1A + b_2B + b_3C + b_{12}AB + b_{23}BC + b_{31}CA + b_{11}A^2 + b_{22}B^2 + b_{33}C^2 + b_{123}ABC \qquad (6.1)$$

The estimated coefficients for factors A, B, and C are shown in the equation: where Y is the dependent variable, b0 is the average of the results from 8 replicates, and bi is the estimated coefficient. The primary impacts (A, B, and C) show the typical outcomes of varying one variable from its minimum to maximum values. Changes in the response due to simultaneous alterations of three components were revealed by the interaction terms (AB, BC, CA, and ABC). To further explore non-linearity, we have introduced the polynomial terms (AB, BC, CA, $A^2$, $B^2$, and $C^2$). Response surface plots were used to help clarify the link between the dependent and independent variables. These plots can be used to investigate how different variables influence a response over time and to foretell how a dependent variable would behave for a range of values for the independent variable. New formulations with the desired responses were then generated using a numerical optimization technique based on the desirability approach.

**Experimental design validation**

The experimental values of the responses were compared quantitatively with the predicted values, and the relative error (percent) was determined using the following equation in order to verify the experimental design (Eq.1). By picking levels of variables at random (A

= -0.5 level, B = 0 level, and C = +0.5) (Table 2), a checkpoint batch (ATN-O) was made and all physical attributes of tablets were assessed.

Relative error (%) = [(Predicted value − Experiment value)/ Predicted value] × 100     (2)

## Stability testing

To ensure that the optimised SMET formulations were safe to use, stability tests were performed in accordance with ICH recommendations [12, 15]. Sodium chloride solution (75 percent RH) was used to desiccate the formulations stored in polyethylene bottles [16]. Three months in a 40 degree Celsius oven were spent drying out the desiccator [17]. The tablets' hardness values, disintegration times, and dissolution times were measured at various intervals and compared using a paired Student's t-test. The cutoff for significance was set at 0.05.

## Chromatographic condition

Analyses of ATVN in plasma were performed using a reverse-phase high-performance liquid chromatography system (HPLC, Shimadzu Prominence LC 20 AT, Japan) with a Pinnacle II C18 column (150mm 4.5 mm 5 µm). An ammonium acetate buffer (pH 4.0) and acetonitrile (at a ratio of 58:42) was used to create the mobile phase. At a rate of 1 ml/min, the mobile phase was pumped. This was done by establishing a 248 nm reading with the UV detector (248 nm, Shimadzu Prominence SPD 20A UV/VIS detector, Japan). For the purpose of processing plasma samples, simvastatin was taken into consideration as an internal standard. Atorvastatin and simvastatin had retention times of 8.4 and 11.8 minutes, respectively.

## Plasma sample processing

Using a 2 mL stopper centrifuge tube, a sample of rat plasma was withdrawn in an aliquot volume of 190 µL. This was combined with 10µL of a Simvastatin (an internal standard) solution (100 µg/mL) for 20 seconds. For 10 minutes, the drug was extracted by spinning 1.5 mL of methanol in a spinix vortexer at high speed (4000 rpm, 4°C). We drained off the supernatant and dried it in a nitrogen evaporator. A total of 20 µL of the reconstituted residue was put into an HPLC system for analysis.

## In-Vivo Pharmacokinetic study

The Institutional Ethical Committee at the Gayatri College of Pharmacy in Odisha, India, gave their blessing to conduct a single-dose pharmacokinetic study on SMET containing 10 mg of ATVN (ATN-O) in white male albino rabbits. Guidelines established by the Committee for the Prevention, Control, and Supervision of Experimental Animals (CPCSEA) were followed throughout the studies. Until the final 12 hours before the experiments began, the 1.7-2.2 kilogramme rabbits were allowed unrestricted access to food and drink. Two millilitres of blood were drawn from the marginal ear vein into heparinized collection tubes at 0, 0.25, 0.5, 1, 2, 3, 4, 6, 9, 12, and 24 hours after a single oral administration of tablet (ATN-O) by feeding tube. We centrifuged the blood at room temperature (1000 g) for 10 minutes. Separation of the plasma supernatant layer and subsequent storage at 20 °C allowed for further analysis. The aforementioned RP-HPLC method was used to examine the plasma ATVN levels.

**Calculation of Pharmacokinetic parameters**

Least-squares regression of plasma concentration-time data points of curves defining the terminal log-linear fading phase was used to estimate the first order elimination rate constant ($k_{el}$). Time half-life ($t_{1/2}$) was calculated using $k_{el}$ ($t_{1/2}$ =0.693/$k_{el}$). The linear trapezoidal rule was used to determine the area beneath the plasma concentration-time curve from zero to the last measurable plasma concentration at time t ($AUC_{0-t}$). By multiplying the area by the rate of increase $C_t/k_{el}$ of the area ($AUC_{0-\infty}$), where $C_t$ is the final measurable drug concentration, the area was projected to infinity ($AUC_{0-t}$). The $k_a$, or absorption rate constant, was calculated using the residual approach. From the profile, we learn both the highest concentration of ATVN measured ($C_{max}$) and the time at which this concentration was measured ($T_{max}$). Extrapolating a plot of time over the product of time and concentration yields the area under the trapezoidal rule, which is the AUMC. Using Eqs. (3) and (4), we were able to determine the volume of distribution ($V_d$) and the total clearance rate (TCR). By dividing the area under the concentration-time curve by the area under the concentration-time curve, the average residence time (MRT) was calculated. Clearance (Cl) was determined by dividing the dose by the infinitesimal AUC ($AUC_{0-\infty}$).

$$V_d = (D^0{}_G \,.AUMC)/(AUC)^2 \qquad\qquad (3)$$

$$TCR = k_{el}\,.\,Vd = (Vd\,.\,0{:}693)/t_{1/2} \qquad\qquad (4)$$

**Statistical analysis**

Design-Expert was used for statistical optimization (Stat-Ease Inc., USA). The mean and standard deviation of all data sets are provided (S.D.). There were three separate measurements taken for each variable (n = 3).

**Result and Discussion**

**Drug-Excipient compatibility testing**

When developing a stable dosage form, it is crucial to conduct drug-excipient compatibility tests as a first step. In the DSC thermogram of ATVN, an endothermic peak was seen at 159.6 0C, and this peak was reliably maintained at 159.2 2 0C in the DSC thermo gramme of ATVN-excipients mixes (Figure 1). The formulations were assumed to have no incompatibilities between the medication and the excipients. Furthermore, no changes in colour, appearance, or drug content were discovered after storing drug-excipient blends under stressed circumstances, as shown by the results of isothermal stress testing (Table 1).

**Table 1. Results of IST study of atorvastatin after 3 weeks of storage at stressed conditions**

| Samples | Ratios (drug-excipients) | % Drug remaining | |
| --- | --- | --- | --- |
| | | Control samples | Stressed samples |
| ATVN | – | 135± 0.48 | 116±0.84 |
| ATVN + Oleic acid | 1:1 | 134±0.51 | 122±0.62 |
| ATVN + Span40 | 1:1 | 122±0.43 | 111±1.78 |
| ATVN + Tween80 | 1:1 | 136±0.68 | 122±0.92 |
| ATVN + Cross povidone | 1:1 | 126±1.21 | 114±0.101 |
| ATVN + Maltodextrin | 1:1 | 109±1.28 | 99±1.98 |
| ATVN + MCC | 1:1 | 119±0.89 | 112±1.21 |

*Values expressed as average ± standard deviation; ATVN, Atorvastatin; MCC, Microcrystalline cellulose.

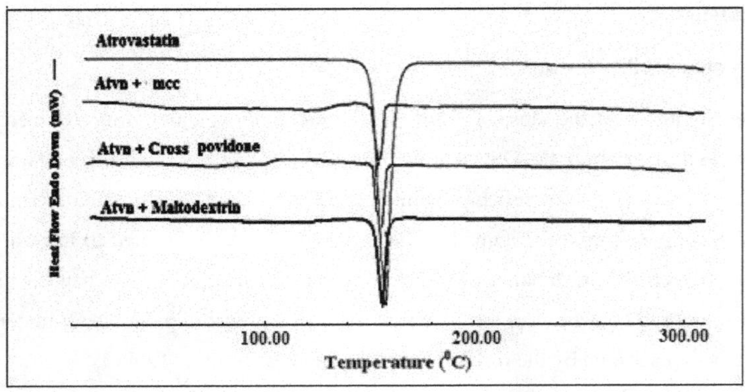


*Atvn, Atorvastatin; MCC, Microcrystalline Cellulose

**Figure 1. Differential scanning calorimetry of drug and drug-excipient mixture**

**Evaluation of granules**

The angle of repose, compressibility index, and Hausner ratio are all useful metrics for evaluating the granules' flow properties. If your Hausner ratio is between 1.03 and 1.08, you have good flow properties; if it's greater than 1.60, you have a problem. All of the produced granules had values of between 21.3 and 25.3 °C for angle of repose, 6.21 and 8.21 percent for compressibility index, and 1.03 and 1.08 for Hausner ratio, indicating that they were free-flowing and suitable for tablet compression.

**Physical evaluation of tablets**

Disintegrating test, hardness, friability, and weight fluctuation were all considered for the tablets. All of the produced tablets had a weight variation of less than 5% (w/w), which is within the allowed range for uncoated tablets according to the United States Pharmacopoeia, National Formulary [19]. All tablets passed the friability test (weight loss 1% w/w), indicating that they had enough mechanical integrity and strength, and their hardness was within the acceptable range of 4–5 kg/cm$^2$. Table 2 shows that the DT ranged from 22.87 1.72 to 86.78 1.38 sec across all formulations, suggesting a rapid pill burst into small globules.

**Table 2. $2^3$full factorial design (coded value in bracket) and formulae with observed response value of atorvastatin self micro-emulsified tablet**

| Name of ingredients | Quantity (mg/tablet) | | | | | | | | |
|---|---|---|---|---|---|---|---|---|---|
| | F-1 | F-2 | F-3 | F-4 | F-5 | F-6 | F-7 | F-8 | ATN-O* |
| **Liquid emulsion Part** | | | | | | | | | |
| Atrovastatin | 10 | 10 | 10 | 10 | 10 | 10 | 10 | 10 | 10 |
| Oleic acid | 10 | 10 | 10 | 10 | 10 | 10 | 10 | 10 | 10 |
| Tween 80 | 5 | 5 | 5 | 5 | 5 | 5 | 5 | 5 | 5 |
| Span40 | 5 | 5 | 5 | 5 | 5 | 5 | 5 | 5 | 5 |
| **Tablet part** | | | | | | | | | |
| Cross povidone (A)** | 50 (-1) | 70 (+1) | 50 (-1) | 70 (+1) | 50 (-1) | 70 (+1) | 50 (-1) | 70 (+1) | 55 (-0.5) |
| Maltodextrin (B)** | 100 (-1) | 100 (-1) | 120 (+1) | 120 (+1) | 100 (-1) | 100 (-1) | 120 (+1) | 120 (+1) | 110 (0) |
| Microcrystaline Cellulose (C)** | 30 (-1) | 30 (-1) | 30 (-1) | 30 (-1) | 50 (+1) | 50 (+1) | 50 (+1) | 50 (+1) | 45 (+0.5) |
| **DT (Sec)** | 58.29 ± 2.19 | 22.8 ± 1.72 | 68.2 ± 3.19 | 33.65 ± 0.87 | 73 .04 ± 2.19 | 28 .16 ± 0.85 | 86.78 ± 1.38 | 40.91 ± 2.38 | 65.06 (Pre) 61.48 ± 2.48 (Act) |
| **$t_{50}$ (min)** | 22.04 ± 3.01 | 6.82 ± 2.18 | 25.32 ± 3.52 | 12.39 ± 2.19 | 27.85 ± 2.16 | 9.69 ± 1.48 | 32.44 ± 3.01 | 15.83 ± 2.47 | 24.66 (Pre) 21.32 ± 3.52 (Act) |
| **$t_{80}$(min)** | 36.32 ± 1.57 | 13.44 ± 2.47 | 39.86 ± 2.82 | 20.31 ± 3.19 | 44.36 ± 1.93 | 17.02 ± 3.28 | 49.64 ± 2.48 | 24.38 ± 3.16 | 38.16 (Pre) 34.74± 2.47(Act) |

*ATN-O, Check point; **Coded Value in bracket

**Particle size and turbidity of oil globules**

When an emulsion sample of SMET was broken up, the resulting droplets ranged in size from 2.73 4.69 to 4.71 6.28 μm. (Table 3). Good emulsification qualities are indicated by the low globule size, as evidenced by a comparison of droplet size data with visual observations. This is because the visual test does not represent the quality of the created emulsion but rather the spontaneity with which it is formed [20]. The same samples that were used for the particle size analysis were also used to evaluate the turbidity (in NTU). Table 3 displays the observed turbidity values in $NTU_{observed}$.

**Table 3. Characterization of granules and self-micro-emulsified tablet**

| Evaluation of granules | | | | | | | | |
|---|---|---|---|---|---|---|---|---|
| | F-1 | F-2 | F-3 | F-4 | F-5 | F-6 | F-7 | F-8 |
| Angle of repose (θ) | 21.3 | 22.6 | 24.2 | 23.8 | 24.6 | 24.8 | 25.3 | 24.1 |
| Compressibility index (%) | 6.21 | 6.52 | 7.22 | 6.18 | 7.51 | 7.83 | 8.21 | 7.18 |
| Hausner ratio | 1.03 | 1.06 | 1.08 | 1.04 | 1.05 | 1.07 | 1.03 | 1.06 |
| **Evaluation of tablets** | | | | | | | | |
| Weight variation (% w/w) | 2.2 ± 1.72 | 3.6 ± 2.64 | 2.8 ± 0.74 | 3.8 ± 1.83 | 1.7 ±2 2.48 | 3.9 ± 1.47 | 4.3 ± 2.38 | 3.7 ± 1.04 |
| Friability weight loss (% w/w) | 0.6 | 0.8 | 0.4 | 0.2 | 0.6 | 0.3 | 0.5 | 0.4 |
| Hardness (Kg/cm$^2$) | 4 | 5 | 4 | 4 | 5 | 4 | 4 | 5 |
| **Evaluation of oil globules** | | | | | | | | |
| Particle size (μm) | 3.08 ± 4.72 | 4.71 ± 6.28 | 2.84 ± 5.18 | 3.67 ± 6.28 | 3.13 ± 8.29 | 4.41 ± 7.29 | 4.28 ± 5.28 | 2.73 ± 4.69 |
| Turbidity (NTU) | 14.31 ± 5.18 | 20.63 ± 4.10 | 24.72 ± 5.19 | 18.28 ± 6.10 | 10.33 ± 4.89 | 28.39 ± 5.39 | 25.04 ± 6.27 | 22.48 ± 5.29 |

**In vitro dissolution study**

Figure 2 shows that when comparing F-2, F-4, F-6, and F-8 with F-1, F-3, F-5, and F-7, the drug release rate from F-2, F-4, F-6, and F-8 was faster and more distinguishable in vitro. This may be attributable to the superdisintegration properties of CP, which were used to their maximum amount (70 percent) in earlier formulations. At 10 minutes, F-2 had the highest drug release percentage (71.43 percent), followed by F-6 (50.45 percent), F-4 (41.67), and F-8 (31.25%). Drug release is reduced in F-6 (MCC, 50 mg) compared to F-2 (CP and maltodextrin amounts are identical). This is due to the hydrophobic nature of MCC (MCC, 30 mg). In contrast to F-6 and F-2, the drug release rate is slower in F-4 (120 mg) due to the complicated network structure of the medication bound to the maltodextrin. The drug release from F-8 is slower than from F-2, F-6, or F-4 because of the higher concentrations of MCC and maltodextrin in F-8. The sluggish drug release from F-1, F-3, F-5, and F-7 may be due to the complex building nature of maltodextrin and the hydrophobicity of MCC. The slow rate of drug release was exacerbated by the greater concentrations of MCC in F-5 and F-7 and maltodextrin in F-1 and F-3. For simple prediction of dissolution data and statistical optimization of formulation variables, the $t_{50}$ and $t_{80}$ values were computed.

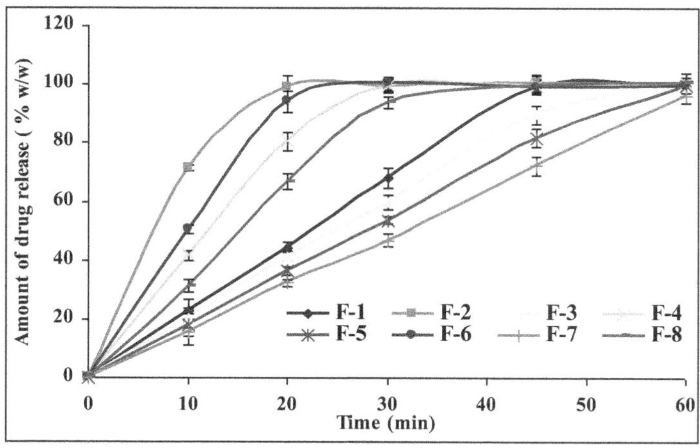


**Figure 2. Self microemulsified tablet of atrovastatin**

**Experimental design and Optimization**

In the $2^3$ factorial design used to create the SMET, each of the three factors, the concentration of Cross povidone (A; 50 and 70 mg/tab), Maltodextrin (B; 100 and 120 mg/tab), and MCC (C; 30 and 50 mg/tab) was given two possible treatments (+1 and -1). (Table 2). Using a quadratic model of the response surface, the standard errors for the independent variables A, B, and C were all 0.354. Concentration of CP, Maltodextrin, and MCC were all investigated to see how they affected DT, $t_{50}$, and $t_{80}$, which are all responses that can be used to determine how well SMET is working for ATVN. Table 2 shows that there is a large range of formulation values (F-1 to F-8) (i.e. DT, 22.87 to 86.78 sec; $t_{50}$, 6.82 to 32.44 min and t80, 13.44 to 49.64 min). The results show that the concentrations of CP, Maltodextrin, and MCC in tablets have a significant effect on the dependent variables of DT, $t_{50}$, and $t_{80}$.

Table 4 displays the results of a one-way analysis of variance (ANOVA) on DT, $t_{50}$, and $t_{80}$ using the selective response surface quadratic predictive approach. To ensure the model's significance and sufficiency, statistical testing in the form of ANOVA was performed. There is a statistically significant relationship between the two variables (P<0.05), as indicated by the model's F value. The probability that the high model F value was due to random chance was merely 0.5%. Model terms are significant if the value of 'Probe' F >0.05, whereas model 'Probe 1' showed that the model test was not significant. Table-6.4 displays the model's significant coefficient. There was a fair amount of concordance between the 'Pred $R^2$' value (DT, 0.998; $t_{50}$, 0.993 and $t_{80}$, 0.997) and the 'Adj $R^2$' value (DT, 0.999; $t_{50}$, 0.999 and $t_{80}$, 0.999). The significance of the coefficient values of polynomial equations was examined. Each coefficient, which might reveal an underlying pattern of interaction between the variables, was given a P value and examined for statistical significance. As the P value decreases, the significance of the associated coefficient increases (P<0.05). Here is the equation that best describes the relationship between DT, $t_{50}$, and $t_{80}$.

$$DT\ (Sec) = 51.5 - 20A + 6B + 5.75C - 2.75AC + 0.75\ BC \tag{6.5}$$

$$t_{50}\ (min) = 19.38 - 7.63A + 2.13B + 2.38C - 1.13AC + 0.63BC \tag{6.6}$$

$$t_{80}\ (min) = 30.38 - 11.88A + 2.88B + 3.13C + 0.63AB - 1.13AC \tag{6.7}$$

**Table 4. Analysis of variance table for dependent variables from full factorial design**

| Source | Sum Square | df | Mean Square | F- Value | Prob > F |
|---|---|---|---|---|---|
| Time require for 50 % of drug release ($t_{50}$; hr) | | | | | |
| Model | 559.625 | 5 | 111.925 | 895.4 | 0.0011 |

| | | | | | |
|---|---|---|---|---|---|
| A | 465.125 | 1 | 465.125 | 3721 | 0.0003 |
| B | 36.125 | 1 | 36.125 | 289 | 0.0034 |
| C | 45.125 | 1 | 45.125 | 361 | 0.0028 |
| AC | 10.125 | 1 | 10.125 | 81 | 0.0121 |
| BC | 3.125 | 1 | 3.125 | 25 | 0.0377 |
| **Time require for 80 % of drug release ($t_{80}$; hr)** | | | | | |
| Model | 1285.625 | 5 | 257.125 | 2057 | 0.0005 |
| A | 1128.125 | 1 | 1128.125 | 9025 | 0.0001 |
| B | 66.125 | 1 | 66.125 | 529 | 0.0019 |
| C | 78.125 | 1 | 78.125 | 625 | 0.0016 |
| AB | 3.125 | 1 | 3.125 | 25 | 0.0377 |
| AC | 10.125 | 1 | 10.125 | 81 | 0.0121 |
| **Disintegration time (DT; Sec)** | | | | | |
| Model | 3817.5 | 5 | 763.5 | 3054 | 0.0003 |
| A | 3200 | 1 | 3200 | 12800 | < 0.0001 |
| B | 288 | 1 | 288 | 1152 | 0.0009 |
| C | 264.5 | 1 | 264.5 | 1058 | 0.0009 |
| AC | 60.5 | 1 | 60.5 | 242 | 0.0041 |
| BC | 4.5 | 1 | 4.5 | 18 | 0.0513 |

All responses are directly proportional to Maltodextrin (B) and MCC (C) concentration, as indicated by the positive (+vet) sign of the coefficient of factor-B and C in all equations (Eq.

6.5-6.7). (C). The reactions are negatively correlated with the CP (A) concentration in the tablet, as indicated by the negative coefficient of factor-A (Eq. 5-7).

Figures 3a, 3b, and 3c display the three-dimensional plots of the regression equation that were generated by the software Design Expert at the midpoint of one factor (MCC). It is hypothesised that DT, $t_{50}$, and $t_{80}$ are directly proportional to B and inversely proportional to A based on the 3D plot of all responses, which indicated that the wire mesh displayed a downward trend at higher level (+1) and an upward trend at lower level (-1).

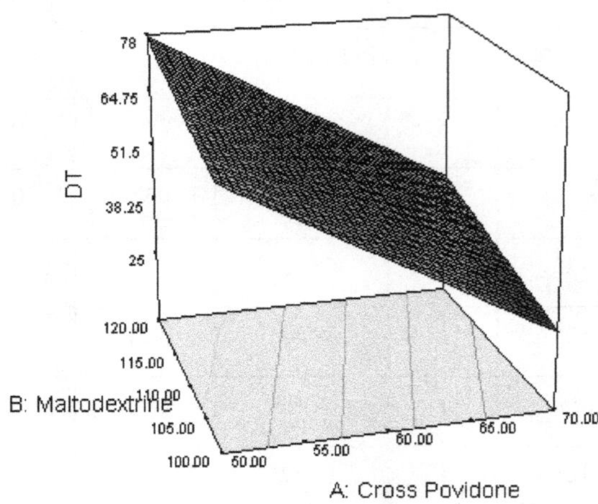

**Figure 3.a. 3Dimention surface plot of disintegration time at 40 mg microcrystalline cellulose**

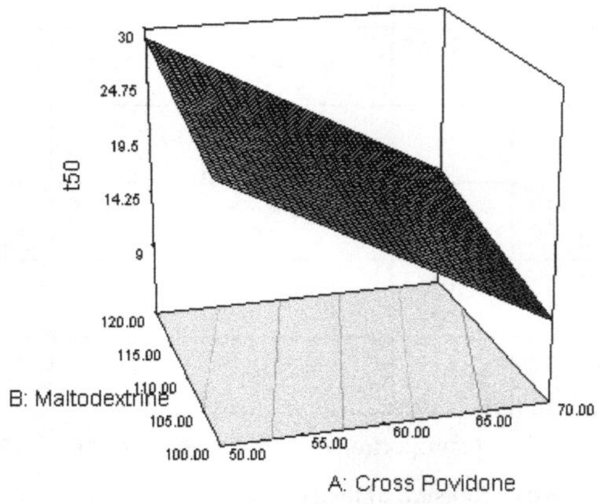

**Figure 3.b. 3Dimention surface plot of $t_{50}$ at 40 mg microcrystalline cellulose**

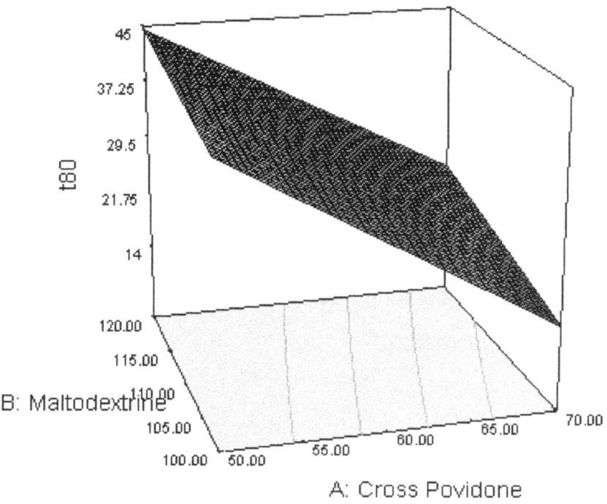

**Figure 3.c. 3Dimention surface plot of $t_{80}$ at 40 mg microcrystalline cellulose**

Graphical optimization was utilised to maximise all answers using a multi-criteria decision-making approach and numerical optimization based on the desirability function at 40 mg/tablet of microcrystalline cellulose (Figure 3.d). By imposing restrictions on the dependent variable and the independent variables, the optimal formulation was produced. Time limits of 23-87 seconds (DT), 10-15 minutes ($t_{50}$), and 25-30 minutes ($t_{80}$) were imposed. All the different formulas shared these restrictions. The Design Expert software used the above plots to determine the optimal concentrations of the independent variables, all of which lie quite close to the 1.0 ideal.

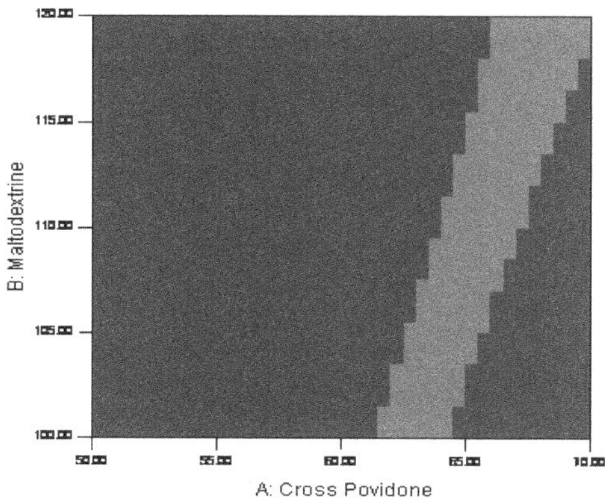

**Figure 3.d. Desirability plot at 40 mg actual factor of microcrystalline cellulose**

**Validation of experimental model**

By picking levels of variables at random (A = -0.5 level, B = 0 level, and C = +0.5) (Table 2), a checkpoint batch (ATN-O) was made and all physical attributes of tablets were assessed. Good agreement was found between the anticipated values of responses, computed from the optimised equation (DT, 65.06 sec; $t_{50}$, 24.66 min; $t_{80}$, 38.16 min) and the actual value of responses acquired from the trials (DT, 61.48 2.48sec; $t_{50}$, 21.32 3.52 min; $t_{80}$, 34.74 2.47 min). This means that all models had mathematical significance, as determined by the outcomes of the statistical optimization method.

**Stability Study**

After being stored for three months at accelerated stability conditions ($40°C\pm2°C$ and $75\%\pm5\%$ RH), the formulations were assessed. Results from stability experiments show that there has been no discernible alteration in tablet appearance, assay ($p<0.05$), DT, $t_{50}$, or $t_{80}$.

**In-Vivo Pharmacokinetic study**

**Table 5. Pharmacokinetic parameters of single dose administration of SMET of 10 mg atorvastatin to rabbits**

| Pharmacokinetic parameters; (n=3) | Observed value |
| --- | --- |
| Maximum plasma concentration, $C_{max}$ ($\mu g/mL$) | $14.65 \pm 0.78$ |
| Time required to reach maximum plasma concentration, $t_{max}$ (h) | $1.17 \pm 0.37$ |
| Area under the curve, $AUC_{0-\infty}$ (hr $\mu g/mL$) | $235.62 \pm 10.95$ |
| Elimination rate constant, $K_e$ ($h^{-1}$) | $0.02 \pm 0.01$ |
| Elimination half life, $t_{1/2}$ (h) | $28.90 \pm 1.49$ |
| Area under momentum curve, $AUMC_{0-\infty}$ ($hr^2$ $\mu g/mL$) | $2601.53 \pm 117.21$ |
| Mean residence time, MRT (h) | $11.04 \pm 0.50$ |
| Absorption rate constant, $K_a$ ($h^{-1}$) | $1.80 \pm 0.12$ |
| Absorption half life $(t_{1/2})_a$ (h) | $0.39 \pm 0.02$ |
| Volume of distribution, $V_d$ (L) | $10.64 \pm 0.73$ |

The bioavailability of the SMET validation batch, i.e. ATN-O, was measured in rabbits to establish pharmacokinetic characteristics. Following a single oral delivery of SMET of ATN-O to three rabbits, the mean plasma concentration versus time curve (Figure 4) and pharmacokinetic parameters have been presented in Table 5. The mean values for the $C_{max}$ and $T_{max}$ of the pill in this investigation were 14.65 ± 0.78 μg/mL and 1.17 ± 0.37 hr. Results showed that the formulation had an $AUC_{0-\infty}$ of 235.62±10.95 μg.h/mL, a $K_e$ of 0.02±0.01 h$^{-1}$, and a $t_{1/2}$ of 28.90 ± 1.49h.

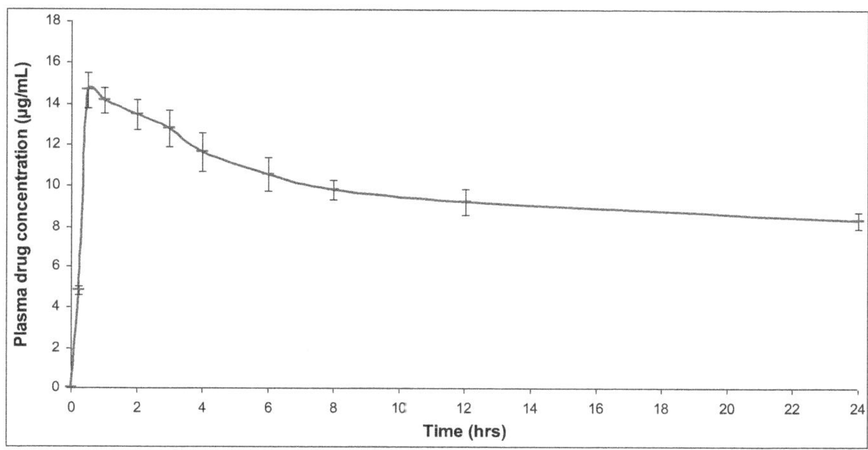


**Figure 4. Mean plasma drug concentration versus time profile after single oral administration of self-emulsified tablet of atorvastatin (ATVN-O) to rabbits**

**Conclusion**

Utilizing a $2^3$ factorial design, we were able to determine the impact of excipients including crosspovidone (A), maltodextrin (B), and microcrystalline cellulose (C) on the disintegration time and dissolve time of atorvastatin SMET tablets. Through the use of polynomial equations, we were able to forecast the quantitative impact of components at varying tiers. All reactions were found to increase in tandem with increasing Maltodextrin and MCC concentrations, and decrease in tandem with increasing CP concentrations in tablets. Predictions of the concentrations of A, B, and C needed for a formulation with the least disintegration and dissolution time value were made using a response surface methodology. Based on these criteria, a revised formulation of the checkpoint was developed. The optimization approach was shown to be feasible in creating self-micro-emulsified tablet dosage forms when the observed responses were in close agreement with the predicted values of the optimised formulation. The formulations were stable at accelerated condition (40$^0$C ± 2$^0$C and 75% ± 5% RH) and droplet size of disintegrated SMET emulsion sample of ATVN was in micron range (2.73 to 4.71 μm). The pharmacokinetic parameters such as $C_{max}$, $t_{max}$, $AUC_{0-\infty}$,

$K_e$ and $t_{1/2}$ of SMET was 14.65 ± 0.78 μg/mL, 1.17 ± 0.37 hr, 235.62 ± 10.95 μg.h/mL, 0.02 ± 0.01 h⁻¹ and 28.90 ± 1.49h respectively.

**References**

1.  Lipinski CA, Drug-like properties and causes of poor solubility and permeability, J Pharmacol Toxicol, 2000, 44, 235-249.

2.  Aungst BJ, Novel formulation strategies for improving oral bioavailability of drugs with poor membrane permeation or presystemic metabolism, J Pharm Sci, 1993, 82, 979–987.

3.  . Robinson JR, Introduction: Semi-solid formulations for oral drug delivery, B Tech Gattefosse, 1996, 89, 11-13.

4.  Constantinides PP, Lipidmicro emulsions for improvingdrug dissolution and oral absorption.Physical andbiopharmaceutical aspects, Pharm Res, 1985, 12, 161-172.

5.  Pouton CW, Lipid formulations for oral administration of drugs: non-emulsifying, self-emulsifying and 'self-microemulsifying'drug delivery systems, Eur J Pharm Sci, 2000, 2, 93–98.

6.  Nazzal S, Smalyukh II Lavrentovich OD and Khan MA, Preparation and in vitro characterization of a eutectic based semisolid self-nanoemulsified drug delivery system (SNEDDS) of Ubiquinone: Mechanism and progress of emulsion formation, Int J Pharm, 2002, 235, 247-265.

7.  Singh SK, Reddy IK and Khan MA, Optimization and characterization of controlled release pellets coated with an experimental latex: II. Cationic drug, Int J Pharm,1996, 141, 179–195.

8.  Spireas S and Sadu S, Enhancement of prednisolone dissolution properties using liquisolid compacts, Int J Pharm,1998, 166, 177–188.

9.  Bolton S, Pharmaceutical statistics,(2nd ed.)1990, NY, USA,Marcel Decker Inc.

10. Pani NR, Nath LK and Bhunia B Formulation,development, and optimization of immediate release nateglinide tablets by factorial design, Drug Discov Therap,2010, 46, 453-458.

11. Pani NR, Nath LK and Acharya S, Compatibility studies of nateglinide with the excipients of immediate release tablets, Acta Pharmaceut,2011, 61,237–247.

12. Acharya S, Patra S and Pani NR, Optimization of HPMC and carbopol concentrations in non-effervescent floating tablet through factorial design, Carbohyd Polym, 2014, 102, 360– 368.

13. Nazzal S, Nutan M, Palamakula A, Shah R, Zaghloul AA and Kha MA, Optimization of a self-nanoemulsified tablet dosage form of ubiquinone using response surface methodology, effect of formulation ingredients, Int. J. Pharm,2002, 240, 103- 114.

14. Carr RL, Evaluating flow properties of solids,Chem. Eng, 1965, 18, 163–168.

15. Stability testing of new drug substances and products.ICH harmonized tripartite guideline.2003.http://www.ich.org/LOB/media/MEDIA419.pdf (accessed Aug 14, 2012).

16. O'Neil MJ, Smith A and Heckelman PE, The Merck Index (11th ed) Merck and Co, Inc., Whitehouse Station, NJ, USA.

17. Patel A, Modasiya M, Shah D and Patel V, Development and in vivo floating behavior of verapamil HCl intragastric floating tablets, AAPS Pharm Sci Tech, 2009, 10, 310–315.

18. Lachman L, Lieberman H and Kanig J, The theory and practice of industrial pharmacy, (3rd ed)1987, Varghese publication house

19. United State Pharmacopoeia, National Formulary,USP, 2004

20. Craig DQM, Lievens HSR, Pitt KG and Storey DE, An investigation into the physico-chemical properties of self-emulsifying systems using low frequency dielectric spectroscopy, surface tension measurements and article size analysis, Int J Pharm,1993, 96, 147–155.